MW00784111

Rhoda Field

"Classified by Common Symptoms"

Meridian Exercise
for Self-Healing Book1

Ilchi Lee

"Classified by Common Symptoms"

Meridian Exercise
for Self-Healing Book1

Copyright©2003 by Ilchi Lee
All rights reserved.
No part of this book may be reproduced
or transmitted in any form whatsoever,
without permission in writing from the publisher.

Healing Society, Inc.
7664 W. Lake Mead Blvd. #109
Las Vegas, NV 89128

e-mail: book@healingsociety.org
Web site: www.healingplaza.com

Call 1-877-324-6425, toll-free.

Library of Congress Control Number: 2003104266
ISBN 0-9720282-7-7

Printed in South Korea

"Classified by Common Symptoms"

Meridian Exercise
for Self-Healing Book 1

Ilchi Lee

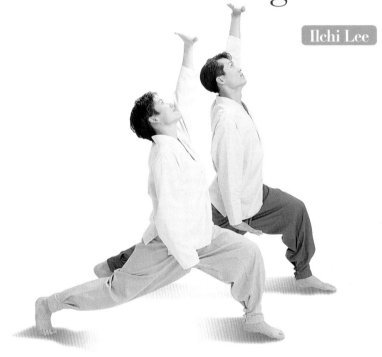

Healing Society

PREFACE

In the twenty-first century, health remains an increasingly important subject. Although cancer remedies, use of hormones to prevent aging and other medical advancements proliferate, there is no sign that incidence of illness is decreasing. Environmental pollution, food and water contamination and stress are taking an increasing toll on our bodies.

It is high time for us to re-evaluate existing medical practices. Modern medicine focuses on treatment, rather than on prevention of disease. Though state of the art treatment is important, making progress in the area of preventive medicine is far more important. Beyond the limitations of pills and surgery prescribed for symptomatic treatment, we need to adopt a holistic perspective and treat the human body as a wholly integrated organism. The human body is an organism composed of interconnected organs that profoundly affect one another. When there is a problem with the stomach, instead of reaching for a scalpel, we should examine and improve functioning of the whole body in relation to the stomach.

For the past 20 years, I have been systemizing and improving Korea's traditional training method, known as Dahnhak to fit the modern lifestyle. Research, clinical testing and practical experience confirm the effectiveness of Dahnhak in the prevention of disease and degeneration. Dahnhak strengthens the body and its natural healing power by strengthening the fundamental life force. Dahnhak Meridian exercise is basic Dahnhak training and is a comprehensive health regimen that expands to enrich the spiritual body as well as bringing health to body and mind.

   Look through the table of contents and identify your particular symptoms. Then find the specific corresponding exercises that you can perform to relieve your symptoms. The exercises in this book not only eliminate painful symptoms, but also enhance overall health to aid in prevention of disease. You may individualize your exercise program according to your particular needs. If you are experiencing specific health issues, it is advisable to consult with a health care professional before proceeding with the training.

   It is most important to experience Dahnhak with your body. The methods presented here will not help you unless you experience them physically. It is through continuous practice that you will experience the benefits of Dahnhak!

Ilchi Lee

CONTENTS

BOOK 1

PREFACE

CHAPTER 1. PREPARATION

1. What is Meridian Exercise ·········· 10
2. Method of Meridian Exercise ······ 12
3. Benefits of Meridian Exercise ······ 14
4. Health Principles ······················· 15
5. Dahn-jon Breathing ···················· 16
6. Hang-gong ······························· 18
7. How to Use This Book ·············· 19

CHAPTER 2. BASIC MERIDIAN
EXERCISE

1. Body Tapping ·················· 22
2. Circulation Exercise ············ 26
3. Dahn-jon Tapping ··············· 27
4. Intestinal Exercise ··············· 28
5. Anal Contracting Exercise ·········· 29

CHAPTER 3. MERIDIAN EXERCISES
FOR SPECIFIC SYMPTOMS

1. BRAIN AND NERVOUS SYSTEM

1) Headaches ······················· 32
2) Facial Nerve Disorders (Bell's Palsy) ········ 42
3) Autonomic Nervous System Difficulties ··· 46
4) Tingling/Numbness in the Hands and Feet 54

2. ENDOCRINE SYSTEM

1) Thyroid Disorders ·············· 58
2) Diabetes ······················· 70

3. RESPIRATORY SYSTEM

1) Lung Disease ···················· 80
2) Cold/Flu ·························· 90

4. BONE, MUSCLE, AND SKIN

1) Lumbago ························· 98
2) Neck Pain ······················ 110
3) Shoulder Pain ·················· 114
4) Sciatic Pain ···················· 122
5) Arthritis ························ 130
6) Osteoporosis ··················· 136
7) Skin Disorders ················· 138
8) Hair Loss ······················ 148

CONTENTS

BOOK 2

PREFACE

CHAPTER 4. MERIDIAN EXERCISES FOR
SPECIFIC SYMPTOMS

1. HEART AND CIRCULATORY SYSTEM

1) Heart Disease ·····························10

2) Hypertension ····························24

3) Hypotension ····························30

4) Stroke ··································34

2. DIGESTIVE SYSTEM

1) Gastrointestinal Disorders ··················38

2) Liver Disorders·························50

3) Diarrhea ······························64

4) Constipation ··························68

5) Hemorrhoids ··························78

3. URINARY TRACT
AND REPRODUCTIVE SYSTEM

1) Kidney Disorders ······················82

2) Bladder Infection ······················90

3) Stamina/Strengthening ·················94

4. EXERCISES FOR WOMEN

1) Exercises for Pregnancy ················102

2) Recovery from Post Partum ···············120

3) Leukorrhea ·······················124

4) Menstrual Disorders ·················132

5. OTHER CONDITIONS

1) Obesity ···························138

2) Poor Eyesight ·····················150

3) Impaired Hearing ···················154

4) Insomnia ························156

5) Hangovers ·············164

6) Lethargy/Fatigue·········170

7) Spring Fatigue ········ 174

APPENDIX

1. The Spine, Main Pillar of our Body 182

2. Position of Organs and the Skeleton 184

3. Meridians, Rivers of Energy 186

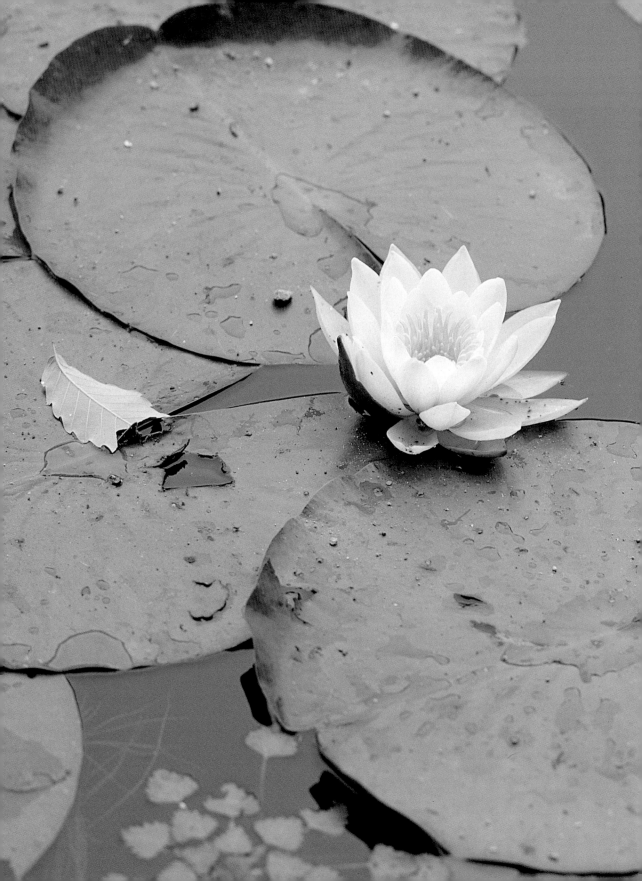

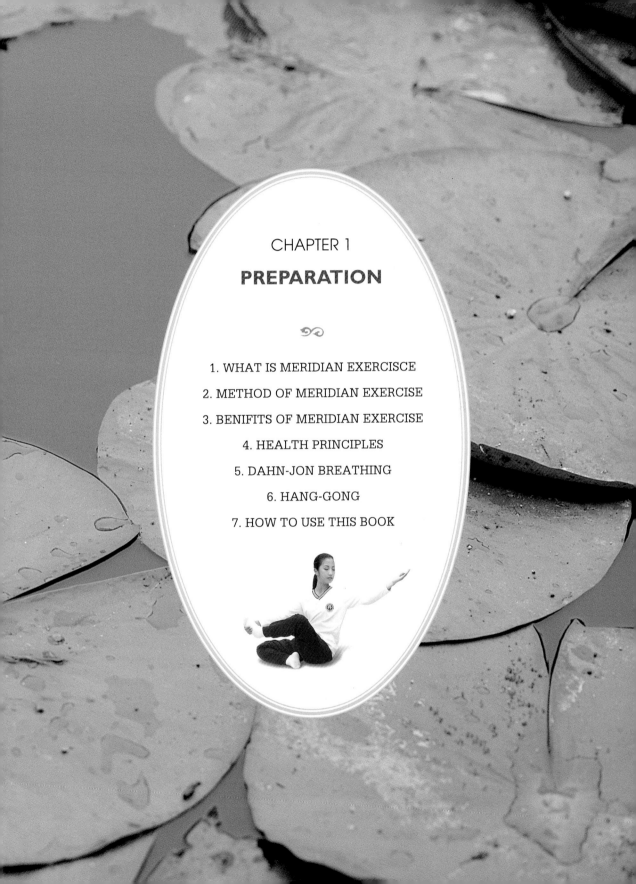

CHAPTER 1

PREPARATION

೨ഌ

1. WHAT IS MERIDIAN EXERCISCE

2. METHOD OF MERIDIAN EXERCISE

3. BENIFITS OF MERIDIAN EXERCISE

4. HEALTH PRINCIPLES

5. DAHN-JON BREATHING

6. HANG-GONG

7. HOW TO USE THIS BOOK

1. WHAT IS MERIDIAN EXERCISE

Dahnhak Meridian exercise is a systematic series of exercises that help the mind and body relax prior to commencing Dahn-jon breathing and other exercises. Pulling and stretching motion of this exercise stimulates the meridian system of the body and facilitates the free flow of energy throughtout the body.

People experience health problems because of blockages in Ki energy and blood circulation. These blockages can result in disease formation thereby weakening the immune system.

In addition, many people evolve using certain parts of their bodies and neglecting others. This results in stiffness and blockages of Ki energy circulation.

People who are young or old, sick or healthy can perform these exercises easily because they are simple and individualized to each person's particular health condition.

The hallmark that distinguishes Dahnhak Meridian exercises in comparison to other exercise modalities, is the trinity of breathing, motion, and consciousness.

As we inhale, the cosmic, fresh Ki energy circulates throughout the body. When we exhale, accumulated toxins in the body are dissipated. Practitioners reports experiencing Ki energy circulation with greater intensity and have an increased sense of well being, peace and joy, along with deeper levels of consciousness and ability to monitor their bodies on their own.

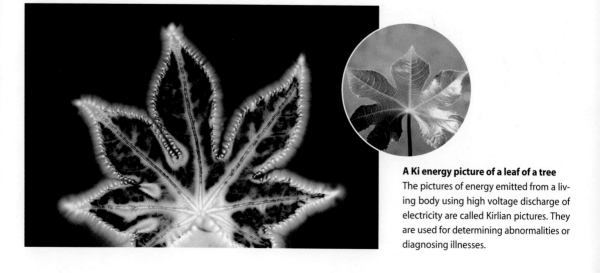

A Ki energy picture of a leaf of a tree
The pictures of energy emitted from a living body using high voltage discharge of electricity are called Kirlian pictures. They are used for determining abnormalities or diagnosing illnesses.

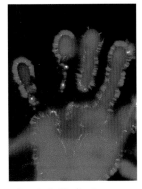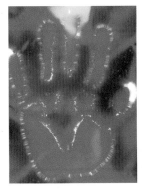

A hand of a Ki practioner

The picture on the left shows a hand at a normal state. The picture on the right shows a hand while emitting Ki energy. You can see that the picture on the right is much brighter and clearer.

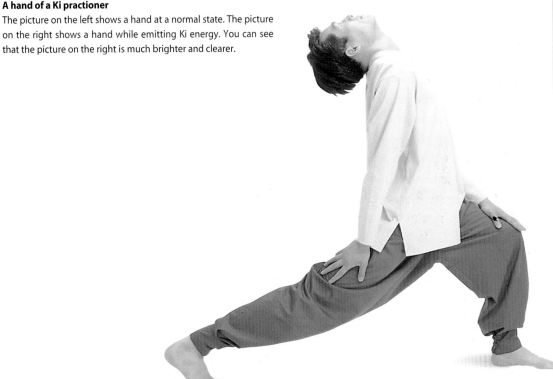

2. METHOD OF MERIDIAN EXERCISE

Meridian exercises can be performed in three ways: lying, sitting, and standing.

When performing the Meridian exercises, each movement will begin with an inhalation and end with an exhalation. Practitioners should concentrate on the Lower Dahn-jon in this process to expedite Dahn-jon warmth and deeper levels of consciousness, signaling the productive Ki energy flow throughout the body.

In augmenting the positive effects of Meridian exercise, the following sequence should be performed: At the beginning of each movement, inhale deeply and slowly while holding the breath throughout the stretch. It is important to simultaneously focus on the Dahn-jon while also concentrating mindfully on the particular part of the body being innervated. This will maximize healing through Ki energy circulation. When you exhale, concentrate mindfully on releasing the stagnant energy that has accumulated in the part of the body you are working with. Then return to the original posture.

If one has high blood pressure, or poor health due to aging, exhale during the stretch.

Perform each exercise very slowly. This will facilitate the opening of the meridians as the stagnant energy or toxins are released from the body. It is important to engage your focused concentration, while progressing at your own pace, rather than comparing yourself to others. Through practice, you can access your own rhythm of regulating your breathing. This will enhance the effectiveness of Meridian exercises. To optimize your comfort, wear loose clothing and be barefoot. At the conclusion of the Meridian exercises, the energy in the room becomes stagnant. It will be helpful to open a door or window in order to allow fresh air to circulate.

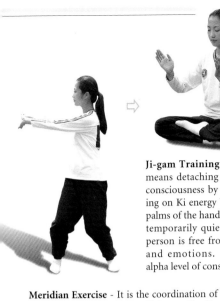
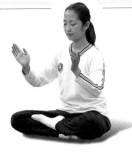
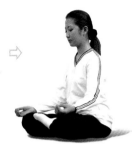

Ji-gam Training - "Ji-gam" means detaching from outer consciousness by concentrating on Ki energy between the palms of the hands. Senses are temporarily quieted and the person is free from thoughts and emotions. Can attain alpha level of consciousness.

Meridian Exercise - It is the coordination of breathing, motion, and mindfulness of bodily movement to access Ki energy circulation. Stretching, pulling, pushing, stimulating the brain, realignment, balance and symmetry of spine; left and right, front and back, and upper and lower. Stimulates and strengthens the internal organs, muscles, nervous, circulatory, and immune systems. The meridian system is activated and cleansed. One begins from parts farthest away from the heart and moves towards the heart.

Dahn-jon Breathing - Purpose is to access Ki energy and bring it into the Dahn-jon through breath, the mediator of mind and body. A holistic, meditative method of respiration. Promotes natural healing power of the body by strengthening the immune system and supporting functions of the organs in the body.

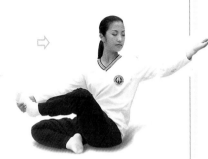

Hang-gong - Series of exercises composed of static postures to facilitate deep Dahn-jon breathing and accumulation of Ki energy in the Dahn-jon. Enhances the ability to coordinate mind and body with relaxed concentration. Fortifies the meridian system and enhances the body's self-healing mechanisms.

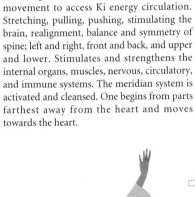
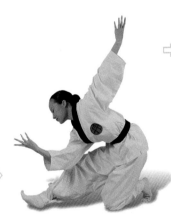
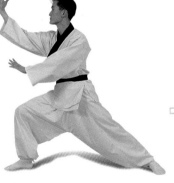

Dahn-mu - "Dahn" means "Ki energy." "Mu" means "dance." The dance of Ki energy. Self-expressive motion is created, with natural Ki energy flow. One lets the Ki energy move one's body. Brings experience of peaceful joy and spontaneity. Self-healing process that stimulates energy centers and meridians.

Dahn-gong - "Dahn" means "Ki Energy." "Gong" means "Martial Arts." Dahn-gong is an advanced level of martial arts developing from the outflow of Ki energy accumulated through practice of Dahn-mu. Ki is stimulated throughout the body.
Acupressure points and meridians are open. Physical and mental health stamina are improved. The mind becomes attuned and synchronized as Ki is cultivated and accumulated. Comprised of five forms, which stimulate different patterns of Ki energy circulation.

BASIC DAHNHAK PRACTICE

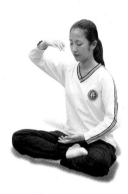

Un-ki-shim-gong - "Un" means "circulation." "Ki" means "energy." "Shim" means "consciousness" and "Gong" means "art." One can consciously control Ki energy through extremely slow and relaxed movements of the arms and hands.
Practitioners can relax and focus on peace, joy and positive attitude, along with deep insight as they reach expanded levels of consciousness. Acupressure points are activated, allowing optimal Ki energy circulation. Composed of nine levels.

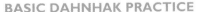

3. BENEFITS OF MERIDIAN EXERCISE

Physical Benefits

- Spine is lengthened and stretched. Height can be increased by 1inch.
- Practitioner develops a keen sense of awareness in distinguishing parts of the body where Ki energy has become blocked .
- Flexibility and strength are developed, stress and fatigue are lessened and released. Internal organs are stimulated, with an accompanying sense of vitality.
- Pelvis and spine is realigned, along with the body re-establishing a natural symmetrical balance. Pain in these areas will diminish as symmetrical balance is optimized
- Enhances body's ability to break down fat cells and increase blood circulation.
- Muscular, nervous and circulatory system is strengthened and meridian system is activated.
- Toxins and stagnant energy in the body are dissipated.
- Increased sense of vitality and energy is experienced as Ki energy is accumulated in the central energy center in the lower abdomen. The practitioner can experience a more vibrant projection of their voice.

Tasks of daily living can be performed with a heightened and more robust sense of well being.

Mental Benefits

- The body becomes very relaxed, thus calming the mind.
- Deep breathing is attained, which stimulates circulation of oxygen to the brain. The head feels clear and memory becomes more astute.
- One's ability to negotiate or manage stress is increased, as well as the ability to control emotions and thoughts. Positive attitude and joy towards life becomes intensified.
- When this exercise is performed with sincerity, the practitioner can appreciate the workings of the mind/body/spirit synchronicity.
- The trinity of breathing, motion, and consciousness, that are the hallmark of Meridian exercise, optimizes concentration with an accompanying sense of mastery over the body. This facilitates and maximizes the self-healing process.

4. HEALTH PRINCIPLES

Meridian exercise is a systematic stretching exercise based on the perfect coordination of the correct postures, breathing, and consciousness. It corrects spinal structure by enhancing symmetrical balancing of the spine, and restoring balance in the shape of the body. It relieves stress and fatigue, promotes relaxation and full rest, and releases anxiety. The spinal cord is the central pillar of the bodily structure, and all of the organs are connected to it by the nerve system. Therefore, any problems with the spinal cord will cause equivalent problems in the related organs and disease can occur. Dahnhak practice strengthens and activates the spinal cord by giving it positive stimulation and helps the body keep in shape and balance. There is increased physical well-being, as well as mental well-being, as one experiences an increased sense of peace along with positive thinking and confidence.

Harmony and balance are major precepts for good health. Our body gets healthier when we balance our body, mind, and spirit. Bone, muscle, nerve, organ, and nature are all connected and must be balanced and harmonized. Meridian exercise is a method for creating harmony and balance. By performing these exercises, spinal alignment occurs, and with proper breath, Ki energy is accessed and harmonized with the body. The person feels more harmonized with others and the world (nature) around them. With the synchronization of body movements and breath, Ki energy flows to the organs and major Ki centers to facilitate this harmony.

The relationship between the five organs and Ki energy

Generating sequence (Cooperative relationship)

Contolling sequence (Incooperative relationship)

5. DAHN-JON BREATHING

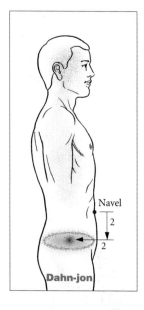

During Dahn-jon breathing, you bring your mind to your lower Dahn-jon and coordinate it with your breath to accumulate energy in that area. You can achieve peace of mind and confidence as you practice this. Dahn-jon breathing helps establish clarity and focus. Dahn-jon breathing is not only physical, but the joining together of the body and mind.

Anatomically, we cannot prove there is a Dahn-jon. Through Dahn-jon breathing, one can experience a certain sensation in the area of the lower Dahn-jon, two inches below the navel and two inches inside the lower abdomen. We have seven Dahn-jons - four external and three internal. Dahn-jon breathing refers to the lower Dahn-jon.

The Korean culture practiced Dahnhak thousands of years ago. I have modernized it. Before modernization, the three methods of exercise were Ji-gam(quiet mind), Jo-shik(control breathing), and Geum-chok(stop contact). In mordern Dahnhak practice, "Jo-shik" is called Dahn-jon breathing .

In Dahnhak practice, there is Myung-moon breathing. This is different from Dahn-jon breathing in that Myung-moon breathing is inhaling Ki energy through the Myung-moon acupressure point. Although you breathe in through your nose, your focus remains on your Dahn-jon and Myung-moon. Regulate your breathing slowly and comfortably. As you inhale, and concentrate on the Myung-moon,

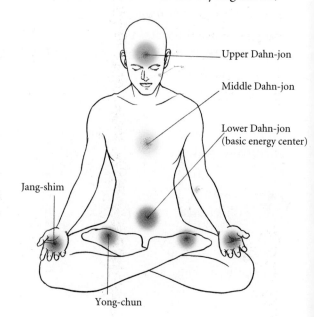

Seven Dahn-jons

the abdomen expands. As you exhale, the lower abdomen contracts, and concentration is on energy exiting through the Myung-moon. Through this process, the Dahn-jon and the Myung-moon become one.

LOCATION OF MYUNG-MOON

"Myung-moon" means the gate of life. The Myung-moon is an acupressure point located between the second and third lumbar vertebrae. The five lumbar vertebrae are located around the waist area. The Myung-moon is opposite the navel. To locate the Myung-moon, imagine drawing a straight line from the navel around to the lumbar vertebrae. Begin with your fingers touching at your navel, with thumbs facing towards the back. Move your hands towards your back along the waist meeting your thumbs along the vertebrae of your spine. They will meet at the junction between the second and third lumbar vertebrae which is the Myung-moon point.

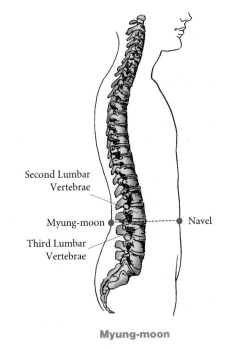

Second Lumbar Vertebrae

Myung-moon — — — — Navel

Third Lumbar Vertebrae

Myung-moon

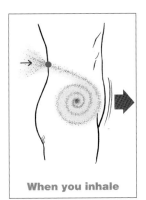

When you inhale

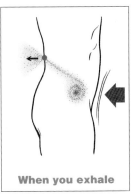

When you exhale

6. HANG-GONG

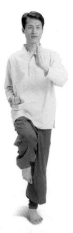

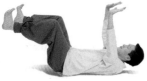

Lying Style

Hang-gong is composed of static postures, which facilitate Dahn-jon breathing. Dahn-jon breathing is utilized with several postures. Moving past the traditional half and full lotus postures for meditation, practitioners deepen their meditation practice by adopting radically different, non-traditional postures. These expanded meditation poses fortify the meridian system and improve the self-healing mechanisms of the body.

Hang-gong consists of nine levels, with five different postures for each level. The flow of Ki energy develops in the body in a similar way to the growth of the human body. Hang-gong imitates the process of a baby lying on its back, turning over, crawling, sitting, and standing up alone. There are different postures that one assumes from three major styles. The first style is "Lying Style". You then progress to the "Sitting Style." Finally you assume "Standing Style." All of these styles utilize Dahn-jon breathing to accumulate Ki energy. With each successive style, the flow of Ki energy increases in the body. The more Hang-gong poses achieved, the faster and deeper the Ki energy

Sitting Style

flows through the body.

If you are a beginner and you try to perform Hang-gong in the Standing Style, you will not be able to accumulate and sense the Ki energy, so beginners should begin with the Lying Style.

Standing Style

The method consists of relaxing the whole body and doing Dahn-jon breathing while simultaneously holding the posture. In the beginning, do five minutes of Hang-gong and then gradually progress to the next levels. In the beginning, it is very difficult to coordinate the holding of the posture, together with Dahn-jon breathing and relaxing. Eventually, with practice you will be able to sense the benefits in your body. Do not force yourself to perform. Rather, attune yourself to gauge your own level.

This book will demonstrate and illustrate various Dahnhak exercises, including Meridian exercise and Hang-gong. You can relieve the distress you feel within your body. Your symptoms will be alleviated and vital energy will increase significantly. You will notice the strengthening of your bone structure and muscles and organs. Your sense of will power and mental capacity will intensify. Ki energy will actively circulate through the meridians with accumulation of cosmic energy at the lower Dahn-jon.

7. HOW TO USE THIS BOOK

The Dahnhak Meridian exercise is different from general exercise. Meridian exercise is bringing positive energy to the body for creative energy. The synchronous movements can have far-reaching healing benefits. If you perform these exercises with honesty and sincerity, you can significantly self-heal the symptoms that cause you distress.

Look through the Table of Contents and identify your particular symptoms. These symptoms correspond to specific exercises you can perform to ameliorate your symptoms. This book specializes not only in healing painful symptoms, but also in enhancing overall health for the body and as a preventative measure. Some of the exercises for certain symptoms will be repeated in different parts of the book. You can individualize the approach according to your particular body condition. If you are experiencing specific health issues which are of concern, it is advisable to consult with a health care professional in whom you trust prior to proceeding with this approach.

The Dahnhak exercises will help to correct the misuse of the body from habits accrued over time. It is important to practice consistently and understand that practice is so very important. Some people want very quick remedies, and thereby become frustrated when this doesn't happen. Dahnhak must be practiced and nurtured over time. You will feel when the condition of your body improves.

As you develop the astuteness in recognizing the nuances of your body's workings, and the skill in deciphering a problem before it intensifies, you continue to progress in becoming an active participant in your own self-healing.

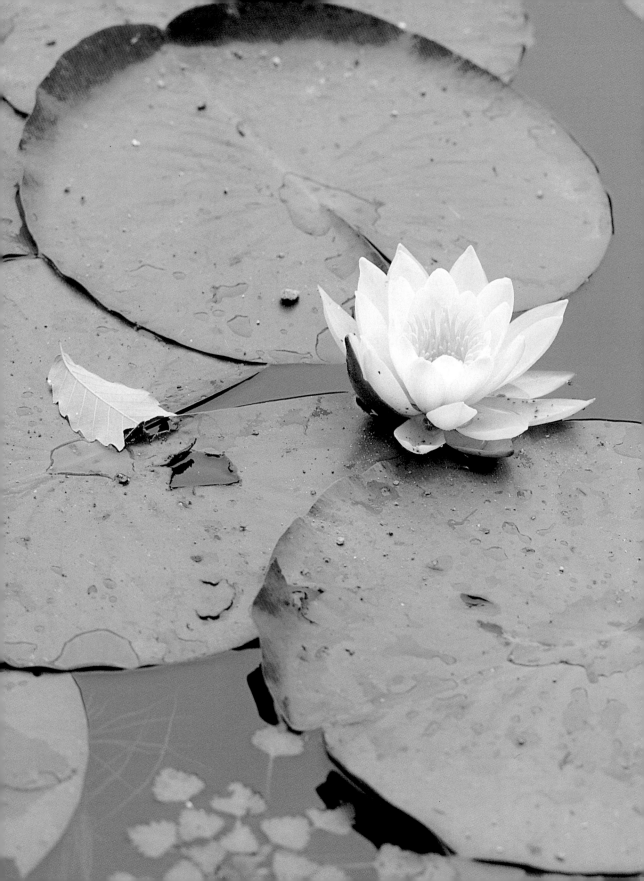

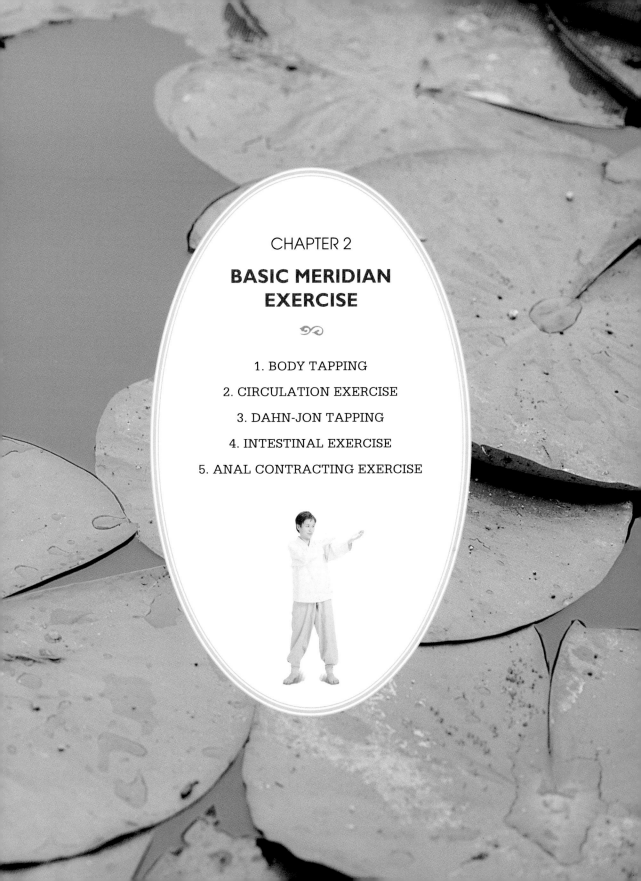

CHAPTER 2

BASIC MERIDIAN EXERCISE

∽

1. BODY TAPPING

2. CIRCULATION EXERCISE

3. DAHN-JON TAPPING

4. INTESTINAL EXERCISE

5. ANAL CONTRACTING EXERCISE

CHAPTER 2

BASIC MERIDIAN EXERCISE

❧

Dahnhak Meridian exercise is a very essential and basic exercise. When you experience tightness in the chest, you would naturally want to relieve it by patting the chest with your hands. If you sense coldness in your hands, you would automatically rub the hands together to circulate blood for accelerating warmth. The Meridian exercises utilize natural body movements. When acupressure points are blocked, you pat them, open them, and get relief. The five methods described here, which could be practiced anywhere with ease, are the warm up sequence prior to doing the Meridian exercises and Dahn-jon Breathing. Daily exercise practiced consistently for twenty minutes will enhance your good health.

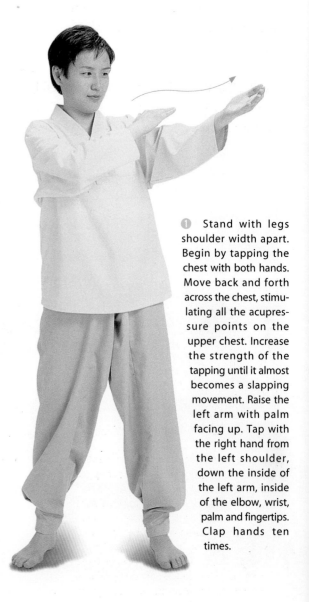

❶ Stand with legs shoulder width apart. Begin by tapping the chest with both hands. Move back and forth across the chest, stimulating all the acupressure points on the upper chest. Increase the strength of the tapping until it almost becomes a slapping movement. Raise the left arm with palm facing up. Tap with the right hand from the left shoulder, down the inside of the left arm, inside of the elbow, wrist, palm and fingertips. Clap hands ten times.

1. BODY TAPPING

Body Tapping consists of tapping the body to help circulation, open blockages, and release stagnant energy throughout the whole body. Through the tapping, cells are strengthened as they are stimulated and acupressure points are opened. All age groups can perform this exercise. It is a very effective method for general health. Tap the body gently and comfortably to achieve the desired results. You can concentrate better if you allow your eyes to follow your movements.

If you feel discomfort in any area of the body you are tapping, do so more lightly. This is particularly important if one experiences stomach distress.

Also, do not press into the area. Instead, gently rub hands together and lightly massage that area.

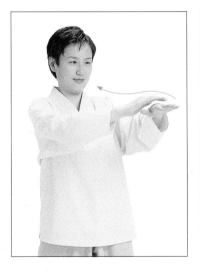 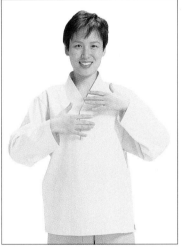 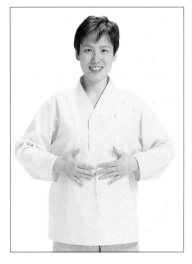

② Then, turn the left arm over so that the palm is facing down. Begin tapping the back of the left hand, up the back of the wrist, the outside of the arm, the outside of the elbow, and back up to the left shoulder. Repeat the same for the right arm. With your right palm face up, tap with the left hand from the right shoulder with the left hand going down toward the palm of the right hand. Then tap the back of the right hand with the palm and then tap up toward the right shoulder.

③ Continue tapping while moving both hands back to the middle of the chest.

④ Move your hands to your stomach and liver and continue tapping.

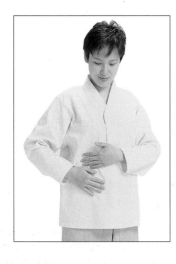

⑤ Pat liver on the right side and concentrate on the liver.

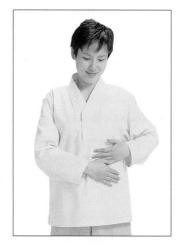

⑥ Pat stomach on the left side while concentrating on the stomach.

⑧ Continue to bend and tap hips and back of hips. Then tap the buttocks and continue down the back of the legs, down to the back of the heels, to the ankles, and the front and top of the feet. Continue to tap upwards from the front of the legs towards the hip joints.

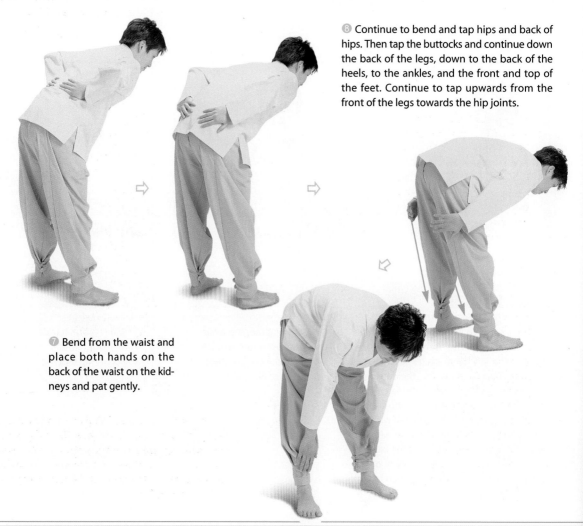

⑦ Bend from the waist and place both hands on the back of the waist on the kidneys and pat gently.

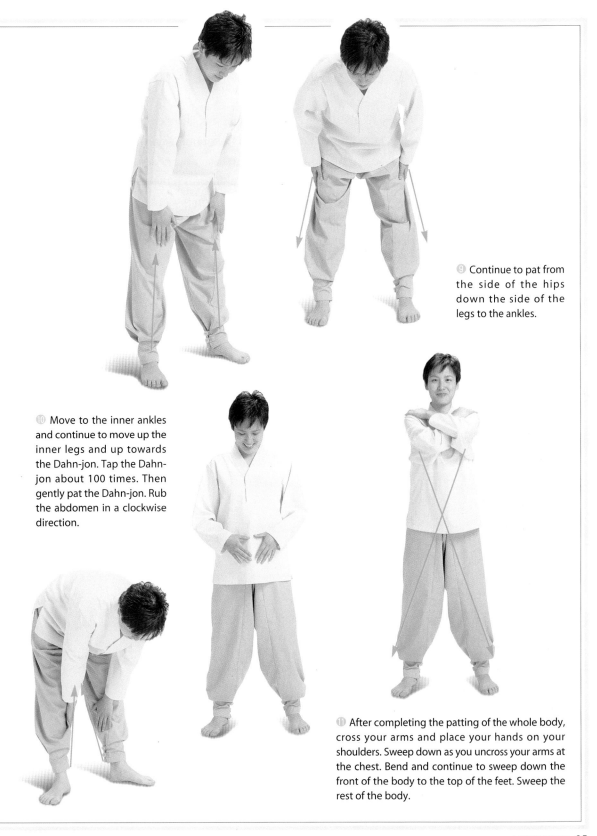

⑨ Continue to pat from the side of the hips down the side of the legs to the ankles.

⑩ Move to the inner ankles and continue to move up the inner legs and up towards the Dahn-jon. Tap the Dahn-jon about 100 times. Then gently pat the Dahn-jon. Rub the abdomen in a clockwise direction.

⑪ After completing the patting of the whole body, cross your arms and place your hands on your shoulders. Sweep down as you uncross your arms at the chest. Bend and continue to sweep down the front of the body to the top of the feet. Sweep the rest of the body.

2. CIRCULATION EXERCISE

This exercise helps to spread Ki energy throughout the body from the Dahn-jon. While lying on your back on the floor, with your hands and feet up in the air, you shake/vibrate your body. This will rid you of tension and stagnant energy. It will strengthen cells and bones from the vibration. The blood in the lower extremities circulates more freely and this helps to slow the acceleration of aging. Also the vibration/shaking, allows for the distribution of oxygen to the brain, which helps brain functioning, particularly concentration, and memory.

Circultation exercise is especially helpful for high blood pressure, heart disease, rheumatism, and bronchial asthma. It helps thyroid disorders and diseases of the skin.

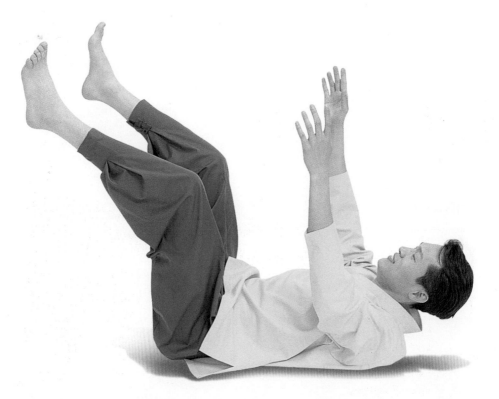

Lie on the floor on your back. Lift your arms and legs straight up from the body, perpendicular to the floor. Relax the body and shake the arms and legs quickly so that the vibration reaches throughout the whole body. Do this for about a minute or two. Rest and repeat five times. If you have any of the disorders listed above, you can increase the time to approximately ten minutes a day. It is important for everyone to practice this daily.

3. DAHN-JON TAPPING

Combined with the Intestine Exercise, the Dahn-jon Tapping Exercise will help the intestines become soft and flexible for Dahn-jon Breathing. This exercise not only stimulates, strengthens, and softens the intestines, but also awakens the Dahn-jon. As you accumulate Ki energy in your Dahn-jon, you will experience an enhanced sense of confidence and well being.

If you eat too much meat, or have poor eating habits, the food does not digest well, causing it to become stagnant in the intestine. This will produce constipation and other gastrointestinal upsets. The accompanying toxins that form will often be responsible for the development of headaches and skin problems as well. Peristalsis becomes compromised and causes age acceleration. The Dahn-jon Tapping helps to lessen this condition and restore normal peristaltic movement.

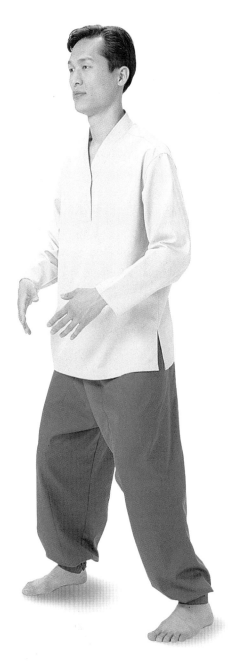

Stand with the feet shoulder width apart. Lengthen and relax your spine. Relax your shoulders, neck, and arms. Bend knees slightly. Place your hands on your abdomen and begin tapping the abdomen in a rhythmic motion with the palms. Increase the pressure of the tapping until it becomes a striking motion. Continue this movement 100 to 300 times. As your Dahn-jon becomes stronger, begin gently and increase the repetitions slowly.

4. INTESTINAL EXERCISE

Proper Dahn-jon breathing will expel the used Ki energy upon exhalation and access and accumulate new Ki energy through inhalation. Dahn-jon Breathing is only effective if the intestines are soft and flexible. Most people, when they begin Dahnhak Practice, have stiff, hard abdomens. The Intestinal Exercise remedies this condition by increasing blood circulation to the intestines and by removing the problem of constipation.

Animals do not become constipated because when they walk, their spines and stomachs undulate. In the standing posture of human, the intestine is pushed down lower and the Large and Small Intestine lose its flexibility and elasticity. In severe cases, they can become strangulated. Because of this, the intestinal walls can form "wrinkles," which cause disease, since food cannot be absorbed and digested properly. With this Intestinal Exercise, peristalsis improves and disease in the intestines can be thwarted or prevented.

This exercise can be performed in a variety of positions, any time and anyplace. You can sit, lie, or stand. It helps to relieve constipation and helps to enhance the digestive system and sometimes cysts in the uterus can disappear. It is an effective and simple exercise to perform. It is important to practice consistently, on a daily basis.

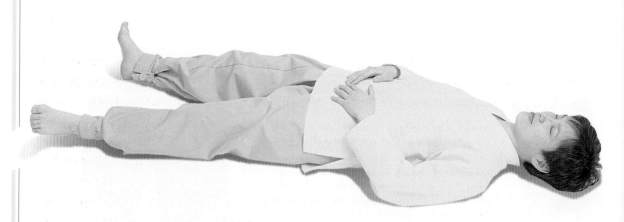

① You can stand (as illustrated on page 27) or lie down on your back. Place your hands on your Dahn-jon with your two thumbs pointing towards the navel and your two index fingers touching together to form a triangle. Push the abdomen out. You will feel a pressure. Pull the abdomen towards the back in an effort to touch the spine. Repeat this movement 100-300 times in a rhythmic movement. Begin gently and increase the repetitions slowly. If there is pain in the intestines during the exercise, stop and gently rub the abdomen in a circular motion, massaging the intestines with the palms.

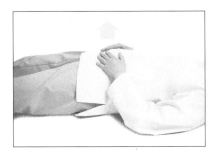

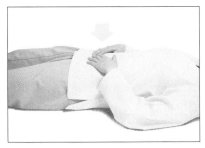

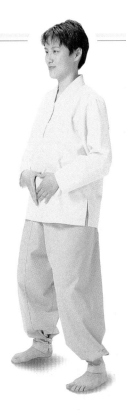

❷ It is best to perform abdominal breathing for more effectiveness. Inhale as you push your abdomen out, and exhale as you contract your abdomen. Hold each inhalation and exhalation for about 2-3 seconds. As you become more proficient at this, you can increase the number of repetitions.

5. ANAL CONTRACTING EXERCISE

This exercise helps stimulate the perineal area. When you sit for long periods of time, feel weak, or have a bloated stomach, the perineal/rectal area loses its elasticity. This can cause hemorrhoids, constipation, and various sexual disorders.

Method　First inhale and hold while contracting your anus, all the way to the navel. Squeeze and tighten buttocks as well. When you exhale, relax the muscles you have contracted. You could perform this without the controlled abdominal breathing, if you prefer.

Benefits　Prevents and heals hemorrhoids vaginal itchiness, as well as bladder, urethra, uterine, prostate, reproductive, and urinary tract disorders. If acute inflammation arises, this exercise is extremely effective. It also aids in the prevention of uterine and prostate cancer. It prevents kidney disease and colon cancer. It also prevents incontinence in bowel and bladder. This exercise helps impotence and erectile disorders in men. It helps maintain and improve elasticity in the vaginal area, thereby helping female sexual disorders. It helps promote healthy sexual relationships.

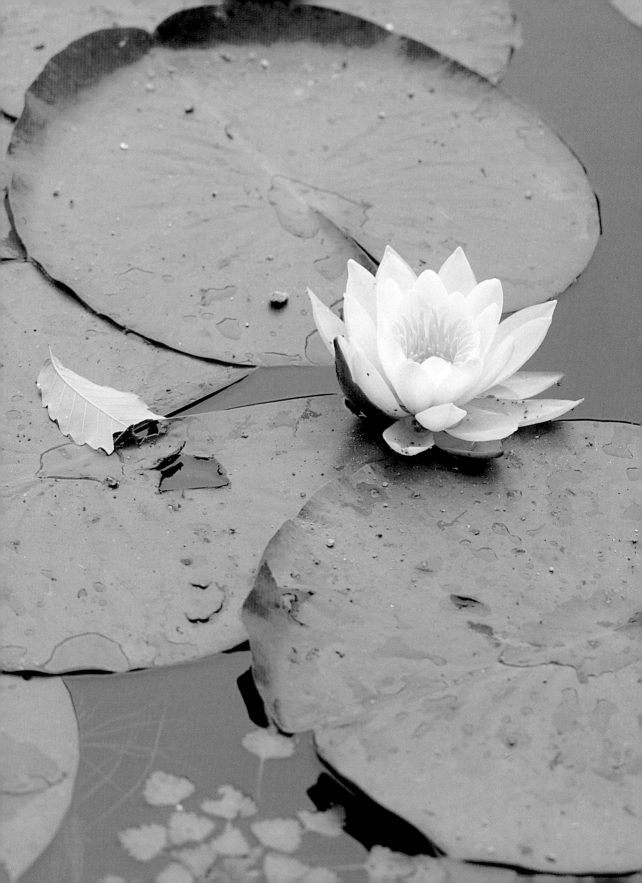

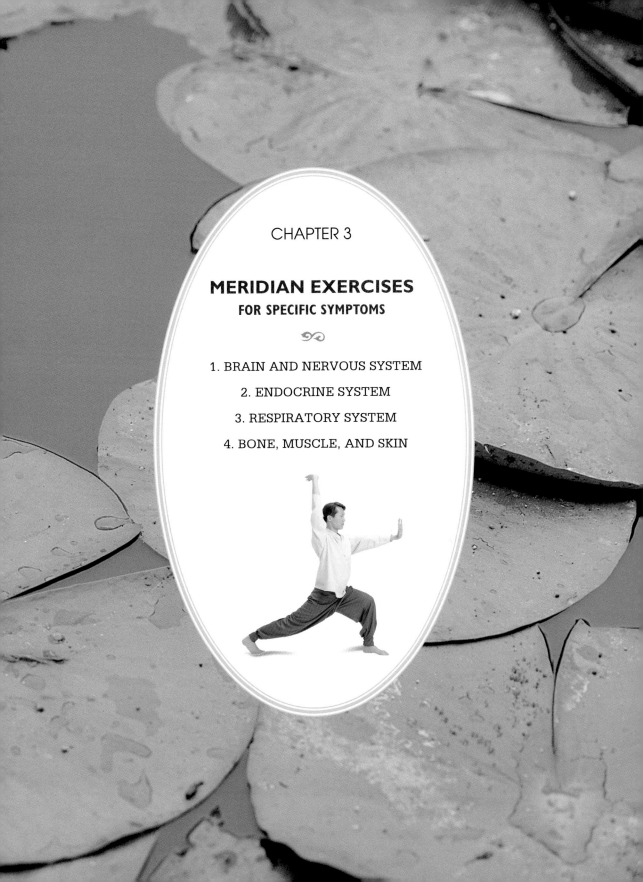

CHAPTER 3

MERIDIAN EXERCISES
FOR SPECIFIC SYMPTOMS

಄

1. BRAIN AND NERVOUS SYSTEM

2. ENDOCRINE SYSTEM

3. RESPIRATORY SYSTEM

4. BONE, MUSCLE, AND SKIN

1) HEADACHES

Like the body's circulatory system, which flows through veins and arteries, Ki energy moves through the body along pathways called meridians or channels. Located on the meridians are specific points called acupressure points. The acupressure points are like openings through which Ki energy enters and exits the body with the breath. Upon inhalation, the flow of the Ki energy enters the body at the acupressure points and moves through the meridians to the vital organs of the body. There are 12 primary meridians and 365 primary acupressure points in the human body.

The Im-maek(Conception Meridian) is the energy channel beginning at the lower lip flowing through the center of the abdomen and to the perineum. When the body signals accelerated conditions of stress, the Im-maek becomes blocked. As people sense this discomfort in their chest, they naturally put their hands on their chest and pat it to relieve the tension there.

The Dok-maek(Governor Meridian) is another of the three major meridians through which Ki energy is circulated. It begins at the perineum, goes up the spine and the top of the head and ends at the upper lip.

The Dae-maek(Girdle Meridian) is the energy channel around the waist beginning at the navel.

There are two kinds of energy in the body: warm fire energy and cold water energy. When the body is in balance and optimum health is achieved, the water energy is located in the head and the fire energy is maintained in the abdomen.

This state is called "Su-Seung-Hwa-Gang." "Su" means "water, "Seung" means "go up," "Hwa" means "fire," and "Gang" means "come down." "Su-Seung-Hwa-Gang" expresses the universal principle that water energy must go up and fire energy must come down.

"Su-Seung-Hwa-Gang" is the universal principle for the life activity in both nature and the human body. In the human body, the water energy is created in the kidneys and the fire energy is produced in the heart. When the water energy moves up through the Dok-maek located in the middle of the back, the brain feels fresh and cool. The fire energy passing through the Im-maek located in the middle of the chest down into the abdomen keeps the intestines warm. After restoring the body back into balance through the Dahnhak Practice, "Su-Seung-Hwa-Gang" is the natural state of a healthy body.

One sign that the body is in balance begins with tasting the saliva in the mouth. If it is sweet and fragrant, the body is in a state of "Su-Seung-Hwa-Gang." Another sign that the body is in balance is when the brain remains cool and fresh while the abdomen is warm and the intestines are working smoothly. The body is refreshed and energized.

A sign that the energy flow is reversed and the fire energy has become stagnant in the head is an occurrence of a headache. Then, the head feels hot and the body feels tired. The mouth feels dry and tastes bitter. The heart may feel heavy and beat irregularly. In this state, one feels tired, anxious, and uncomfortable. Shoulders and neck are stiff. This usually happens after a period of working or studying without moving around. "Su-Seung-Hwa-Gang" is achieved through Dahn-jon Breathing, which expels the used Ki energy upon exhalation and accesses and accumulates new Ki energy through inhalation. Dahn-jon Breathing exercise is only effective if the intestines are soft and flexible. Most people, when they begin Dahnhak practice, have stiff, hard abdomens. The Intestinal Exercise remedies this condition by increasing the blood circulation to the intestines and by removing the problem of constipation.

The following exercises are also effective in ameliorating headaches.

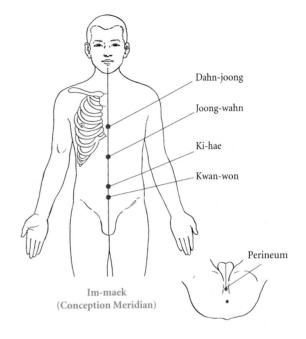

Im-maek
(Conception Meridian)

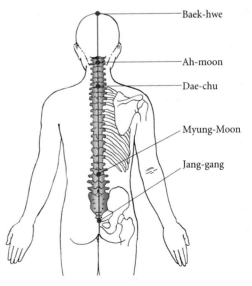

Dok-maek(Governor Meridian)

1. PRESSING THE CHUN-JU ACUPRESSURE POINTS

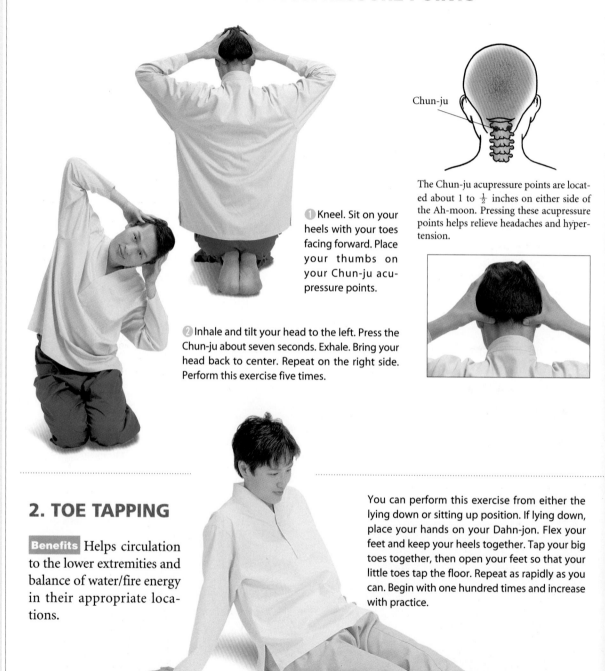

Chun-ju

The Chun-ju acupressure points are located about 1 to $\frac{1}{2}$ inches on either side of the Ah-moon. Pressing these acupressure points helps relieve headaches and hypertension.

❶ Kneel. Sit on your heels with your toes facing forward. Place your thumbs on your Chun-ju acupressure points.

❷ Inhale and tilt your head to the left. Press the Chun-ju about seven seconds. Exhale. Bring your head back to center. Repeat on the right side. Perform this exercise five times.

2. TOE TAPPING

Benefits Helps circulation to the lower extremities and balance of water/fire energy in their appropriate locations.

You can perform this exercise from either the lying down or sitting up position. If lying down, place your hands on your Dahn-jon. Flex your feet and keep your heels together. Tap your big toes together, then open your feet so that your little toes tap the floor. Repeat as rapidly as you can. Begin with one hundred times and increase with practice.

3. STANDING ON THE WOODEN PILLOW

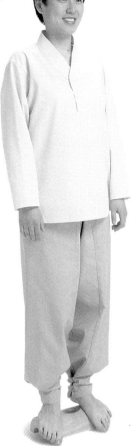

Stand on the Wooden Pillow with bare feet. Face toes towards the floor as much as possible. Massage all parts of your feet for about five minutes as illustrated in the pictures.

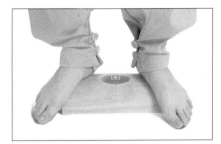

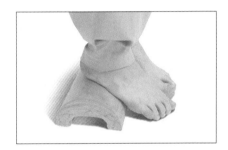

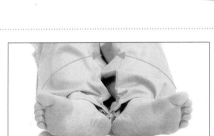

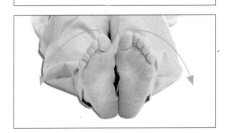

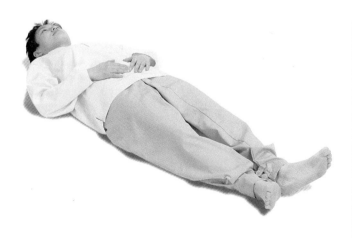

4. HEADSTAND

Benefits Promotes efficient blood circulation to the head and brain-stem. Relieves headaches. Stimulates the brain and regulates hormonal functioning. Enhances memory, concentration, and focus.

TIPS Massage the neck prior to performing a headstand.

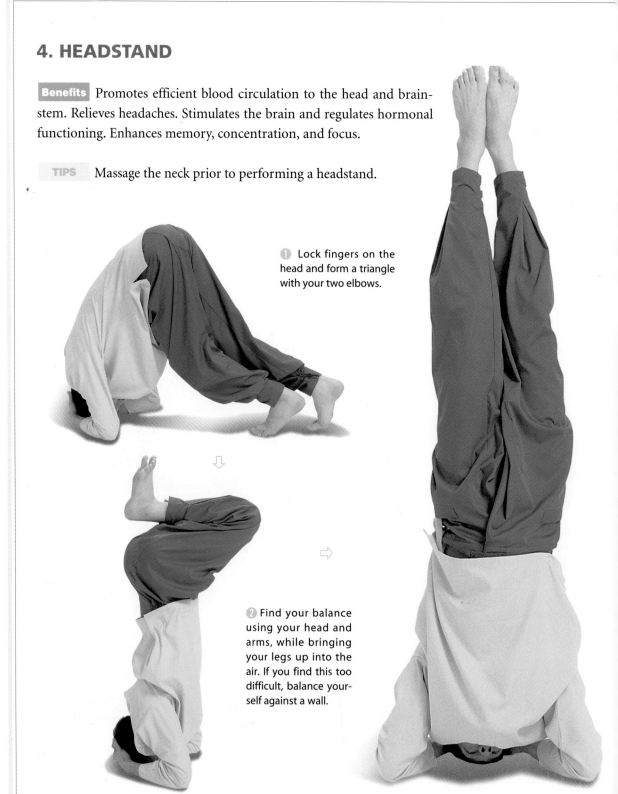

❶ Lock fingers on the head and form a triangle with your two elbows.

❷ Find your balance using your head and arms, while bringing your legs up into the air. If you find this too difficult, balance yourself against a wall.

5. NECK MASSAGE

Benefits When stress is present, the neck and shoulders become stiff and headache occurs. This exercise helps to relieve the headache as you release the tension in the neck and shoulders.

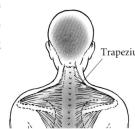

Trapezius muscle

A wide and flat muscle, shaped like a triangle which covers the upper and back part of the neck and shoulders

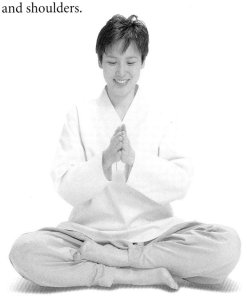

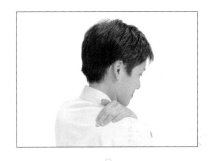

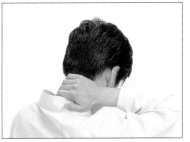

① Rub your hands to create heat. Massage the back of your neck.

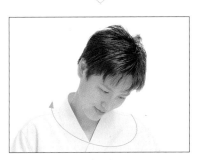

② Rotate your neck to the right and to the left very slowly in a circular motion clockwise and then counter-clockwise.

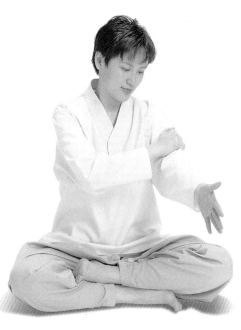

③ Massage your trapezius muscle and then your arm. Repeat with the other side of the trapezius muscle and your other arm.

6. JOK-SAM-NI HITTING

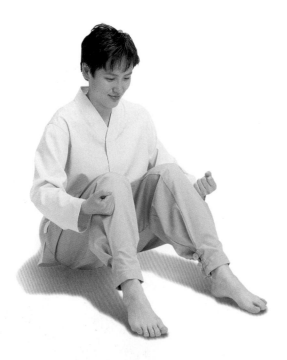

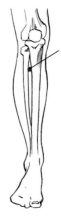

Jok-sam-ni

Located on the outside of the leg, just below the knee, and in between the point where the two leg bones meet. Practitioners of Eastern Medicine believe that stimulating these acupressure points enhances longevity. When you press these points, it helps augment digestion, alleviates headache, circulatory and other problems in the legs, as well as respiratory, cardiovascular, and nasal conditions.

Make a fist without exerting a lot of pressure in the hands. Hit the Jok-sam-ni points one hundred times.

7. PRESSING THE TAE-YANG ACUPRESSURE POINTS

TIPS Do not press strongly on these acupressure points. Press with a comfortable pressure.

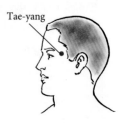

Tae-yang

Tae-yang - Located at the area of the temples.

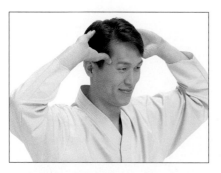

❶ Using thumbs, press Tae-yang acupressure points five times. Do this slowly.

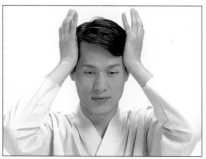

❷ Using the pad of the hands, tap the Tae-yang points thirty times.

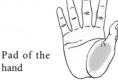

Pad of the hand

8. HEAD STIMULATION

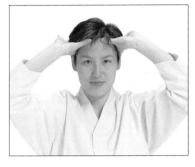 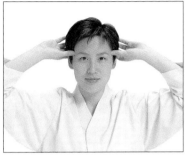 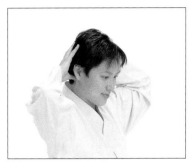

❶ Place thumbs together beginning with the central hairline. Following hairline, move along the circumference of the hairline down towards the back of the neck.

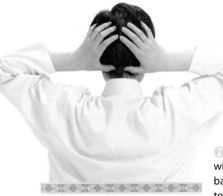 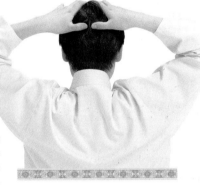

❷ Massage the back of the neck with your thumbs, running up the base of the hairline towards the top of the head. Follow to the central hairline, the starting position of STEP 1. Repeat STEPs 1 and 2.

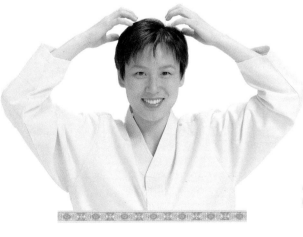

❸ Lightly tap your entire head with your fingertips.

9. CRANE POSTURE

Benefits Clears head and balances right and left hemispheres of the brain. Improves nervous system function and enhances concentration.

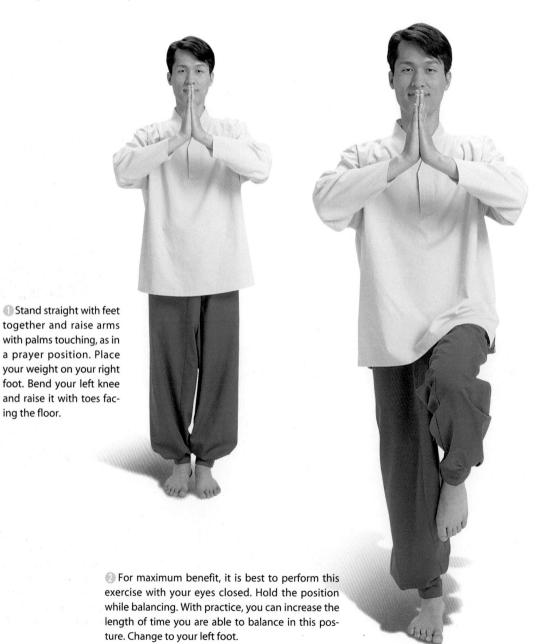

❶ Stand straight with feet together and raise arms with palms touching, as in a prayer position. Place your weight on your right foot. Bend your left knee and raise it with toes facing the floor.

❷ For maximum benefit, it is best to perform this exercise with your eyes closed. Hold the position while balancing. With practice, you can increase the length of time you are able to balance in this posture. Change to your left foot.

10. SOLE HITTING

Benefits The feet are like a "second heart." They are vital in orchestrating proper circulation of the blood. When the soles of the feet are stimulated, brain function is significantly bolstered and you begin to notice a heightened sense of clarity, focus, and concentration.

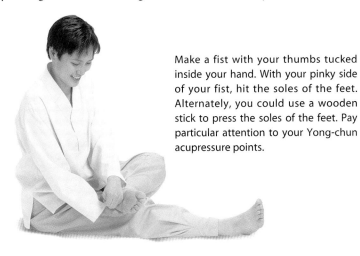

Make a fist with your thumbs tucked inside your hand. With your pinky side of your fist, hit the soles of the feet. Alternately, you could use a wooden stick to press the soles of the feet. Pay particular attention to your Yong-chun acupressure points.

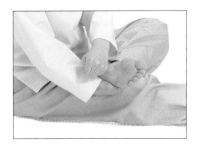

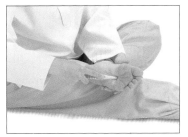

11. FINGER STRETCHING

Benefits Accelerates and increases blood circulation to fingers, which enhances the transport of energy throughout the body. Mental clarity is heightened.

TIPS When you are fatigued, perform less strenuously. When you stretch out your fingers, do so quickly, exerting effort.

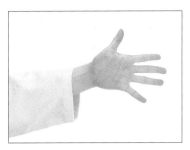

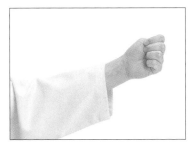

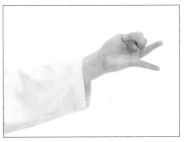

① Make a fist, tucking your thumb inside your hand.

② Open the fist, exerting pressure by thrusting out your pinky finger.

③ Proceed with thrusting open the other fingers of your hand. Stretch them out wide. Go back to position of STEP 1, by first tucking thumb into your hand and closing fist over it as in Step 1. Repeat with your other hand. Perform for thirty seconds with each hand.

2) FACIAL NERVE DISORDERS (Bell's Palsy)

Bell's Palsy is a facial nerve disorder in which there is paralysis across one side of the face. The person experiences weakness of the whole side of the face. The cause is unknown although it is believed that it can occur from exposure to the elements or extreme fatigue or stress. It involves swelling of the nerve possibly due to a compromised immune system or a virus.

When one is able to access the correct acupressure point that innervates the facial nerve, the symptoms can dissipate. If the symptoms have persisted for more than six months, it will be more difficult to treat.

The following exercises are specifically designed to prevent this from occurring. Try to reduce exposure to the cold by covering the area, and minimize undue stress and fatigue from your daily living.

1. PLACING HANDS

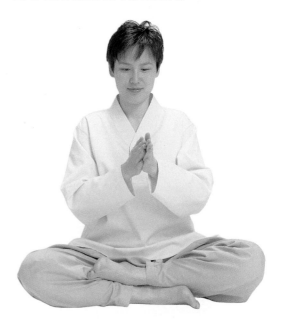

① Inhale from your lower abdomen. Continue to hold your breath while you rub your palms together.

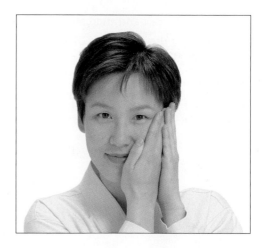

② Place both palms on the Palsy affected area. Exhale slowly. Repeat for five minutes every morning and evening.

2. PRESSING WITH FINGERS TO STIMULATE FACIAL NERVE ACUPRESSURE POINTS

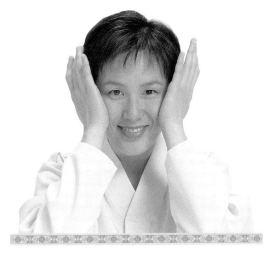

① Place Pad of Palms on your cheeks. Press and rotate. Pay special attention to the area around the mandibular joint.

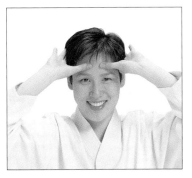 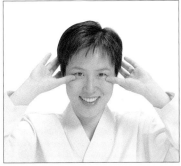

② Place both of your thumbs as in the picture, meeting at the forehead, and begin to rotate them around the eyes.

③ With your index and middle fingers touching, press around the nose, then around the mouth, and proceed to the chin. Spend ten minutes performing this exercise.

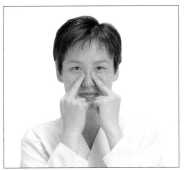 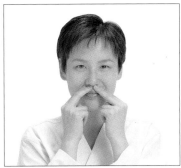 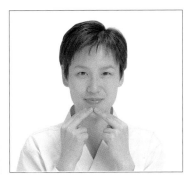

3. HANG-GONG FOR FACIAL PARALYSIS

Benefits Helps facial paralysis and shoulder pain, and strengthens and clears the lungs.

TIPS Begin this exercise by performing for only a couple of minutes. Then progress, with practice to twenty or more minutes a day.

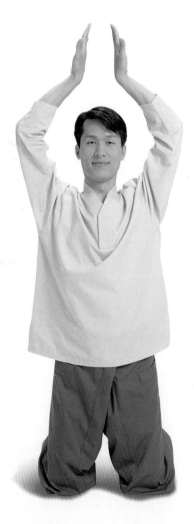 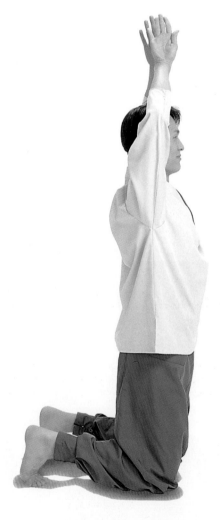

① Bend knees as in the frontal view picture. Toes face forward. Bring both arms above your head, with the back of your hands facing each other overhead. Open your chest.

② Keep your spine straight and breathe normally for up to twenty minutes (see TIPS above).

4. FACIAL MOVEMENT

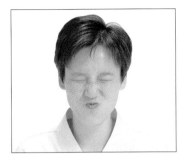
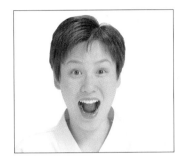

① Contract your facial muscles, including your eyes, nose and mouth. Release with an open-mouthed smile, with eyes wide open, as in the picture.

② Continue to make various faces as shown in the pictures. Look into the mirror while practicing this exercise.

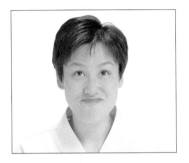
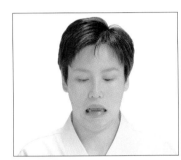
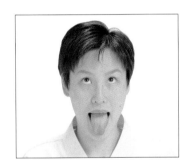

5. CHIN MOVEMENT

Concentrate on keeping your head straight, but with neck and shoulders relaxed, while performing this exercise. Open your mouth and move your chin to the right, as you simultaneously shift your eyes to the left. Then move your chin to the left, while you simultaneously shift your eyes to the right.

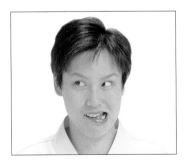
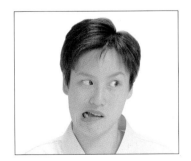

3) AUTONOMIC NERVOUS SYSTEM DIFFICULTIES

The autonomic nervouss system is responsible for the synchronization and regulation of the viscera of the body. This includes the stomach, heart, and intestines. It directs many muscles and organs. For example, the glands of the endocrine system, and the muscles of the eye, stomach, intestines, bladder, skin and heart. The modulation of the temperature of the body is also under the control of the autonomic nervous system.

The autonomic nervous system does not need our awareness to function, since it directs its actions reflexively and involuntarily. However, people can learn to control some of the autonomic nervous system responses, such as the regulation of heart rate, blood pressure, and temperature. In particular, one can control breath voluntarily, which exerts influence on the involuntary nervous system.

Under normal circumstances, there is a balance between the two branches of the autonomic nervous system. However, if the body is continually stressed due to the perception of threats to its well-being, The sympathetic nervous system component of the autonomic nervous system is innervated. In this case, the body prepares for this threat with such things as increases in metabolic rate, heart rate, breathing rate, blood pressure, tension in the muscles, and slowing of digestion. The imbalance that is created here is due to over action of the sympathetic nervous system. If this continues consistently over time, this imbalance of the autonomic nervous system can create disease which begins with such symptoms as fatigue, lack of desire, perspiration, body temperature irregularity, insomnia and other sleep related difficulties, palpitations, tightness in the chest and throat, impotency in males and sexual problems with females, and infertility problems, just to mention a few.

The parasympathetic nervous system branch of the autonomic nervous system is noted for its diminution of sympathetic nervous system activity, which results in a relaxation response. Here we see decreases in metabolism, heart rate, blood pressure, breathing rate, tension in the muscles, and, and increased digestive function.

Through the following exercises, people can exert conscious control over some of the autonomic nervous system functions and create a more harmonious balance between stress, induced by an overactive sympathetic nervous system and relaxation responses accessed through the parasympathetic nervous system. Through postures and breath work, the Dahnhak system demonstrated in this book aims to enhance parasympathetic responses and re-balance and harmonize the two autonomic nervous system branches, thus creating a sense of well being and optimal health.

1. PENDULUM SWING

Benefits This exercise helps to release stagnant energy from the upper body as well as strengthen and enhance the balancing of the autonomic nervous system.

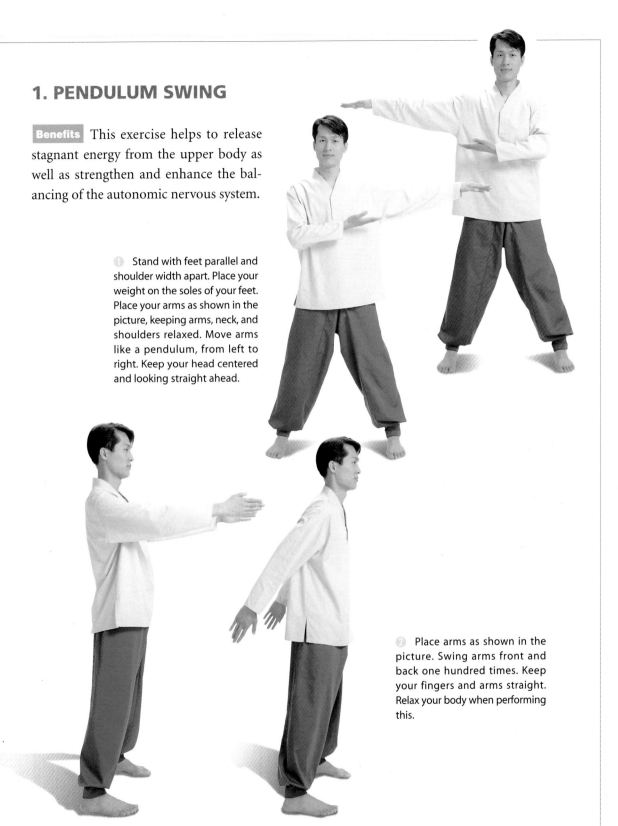

① Stand with feet parallel and shoulder width apart. Place your weight on the soles of your feet. Place your arms as shown in the picture, keeping arms, neck, and shoulders relaxed. Move arms like a pendulum, from left to right. Keep your head centered and looking straight ahead.

② Place arms as shown in the picture. Swing arms front and back one hundred times. Keep your fingers and arms straight. Relax your body when performing this.

2. TIGER FEET POSTURE

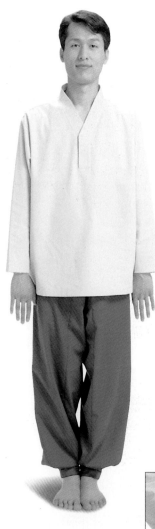

① Stand with feet together with arms at your sides and palms facing toward your back.

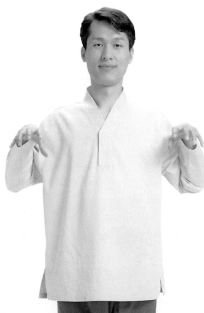

③ Inhale. Raise your hands to chest level.

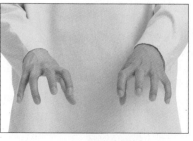

② Imagine holding the mouth of a jar with your hands, with your wrists bent and fingers spread apart, creating tension in your hands.

3. MOVING A JAR

TIPS Concentrate on your spine while performing this movement.

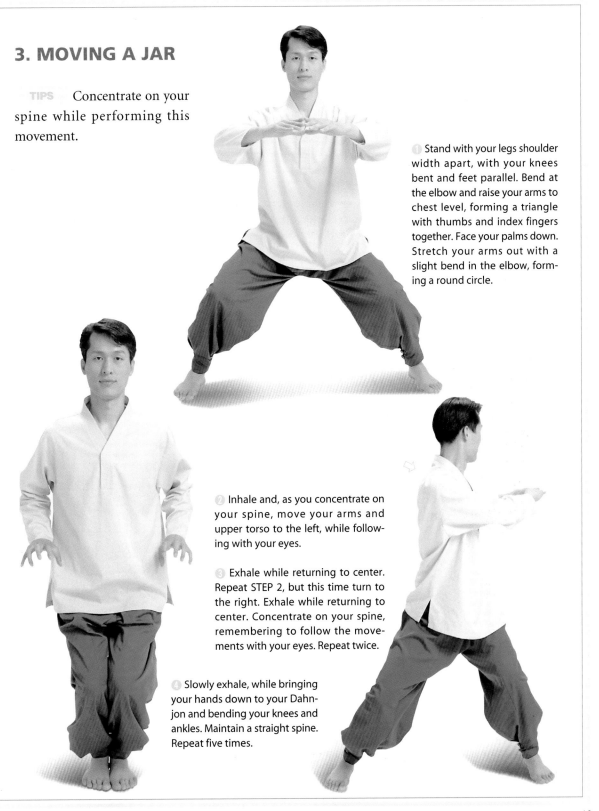

1 Stand with your legs shoulder width apart, with your knees bent and feet parallel. Bend at the elbow and raise your arms to chest level, forming a triangle with thumbs and index fingers together. Face your palms down. Stretch your arms out with a slight bend in the elbow, forming a round circle.

2 Inhale and, as you concentrate on your spine, move your arms and upper torso to the left, while following with your eyes.

3 Exhale while returning to center. Repeat STEP 2, but this time turn to the right. Exhale while returning to center. Concentrate on your spine, remembering to follow the movements with your eyes. Repeat twice.

4 Slowly exhale, while bringing your hands down to your Dahnjon and bending your knees and ankles. Maintain a straight spine. Repeat five times.

4. UPPER BODY LIFT

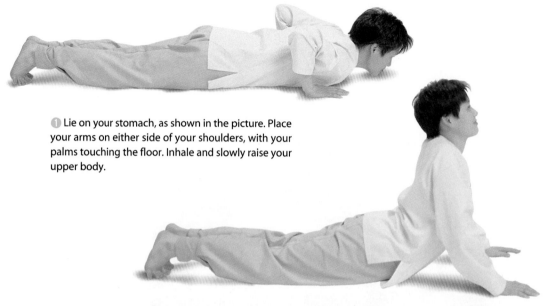

① Lie on your stomach, as shown in the picture. Place your arms on either side of your shoulders, with your palms touching the floor. Inhale and slowly raise your upper body.

② As you raise your upper body, raise your head up and hold it in this position, while concentrating on your spine.

③ Exhale and return to STEP 1. Repeat three times.

5. HEAD STIMULATION

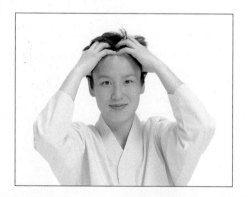

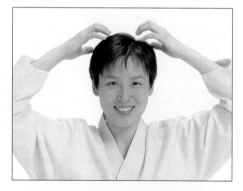

① Place your hands on your head with your fingers apart. Beginning at the forehead, comb with your fingers throughout your scalp area, moving towards the back of the head. Repeat thirty-six times.

② Tap the circumference of your head with your fingers. Smile while performing this.

6. BACK BEND FOR OPENING THE CHEST

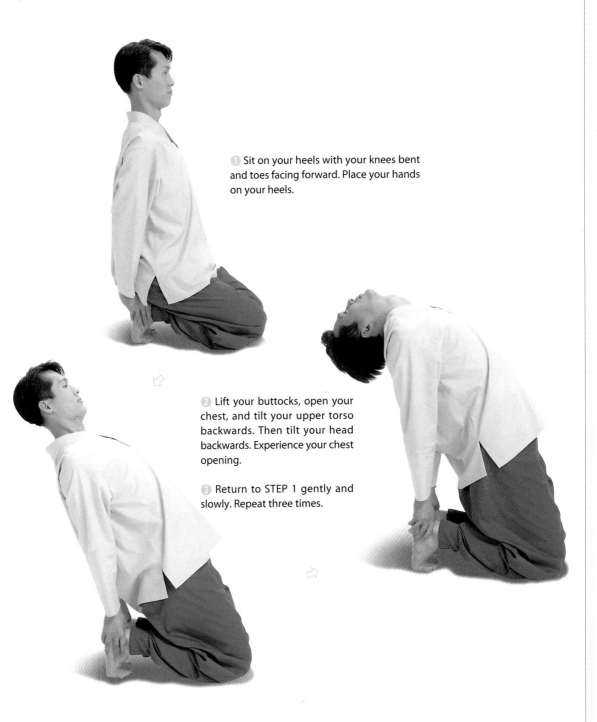

1 Sit on your heels with your knees bent and toes facing forward. Place your hands on your heels.

2 Lift your buttocks, open your chest, and tilt your upper torso backwards. Then tilt your head backwards. Experience your chest opening.

3 Return to STEP 1 gently and slowly. Repeat three times.

7. SITTING FORWARD BEND

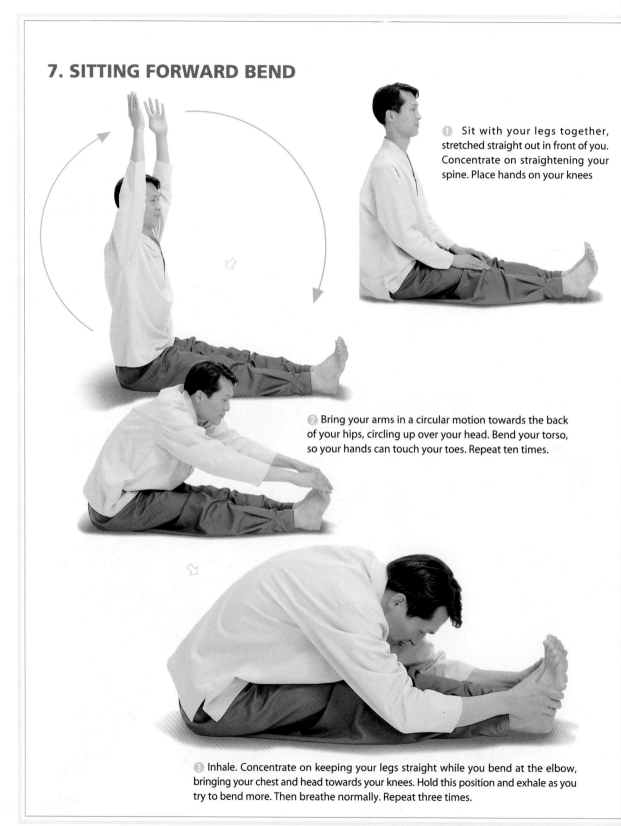

❶ Sit with your legs together, stretched straight out in front of you. Concentrate on straightening your spine. Place hands on your knees

❷ Bring your arms in a circular motion towards the back of your hips, circling up over your head. Bend your torso, so your hands can touch your toes. Repeat ten times.

❸ Inhale. Concentrate on keeping your legs straight while you bend at the elbow, bringing your chest and head towards your knees. Hold this position and exhale as you try to bend more. Then breathe normally. Repeat three times.

8. STRADDLE WITH FORWARD BEND AND HIP LIFT

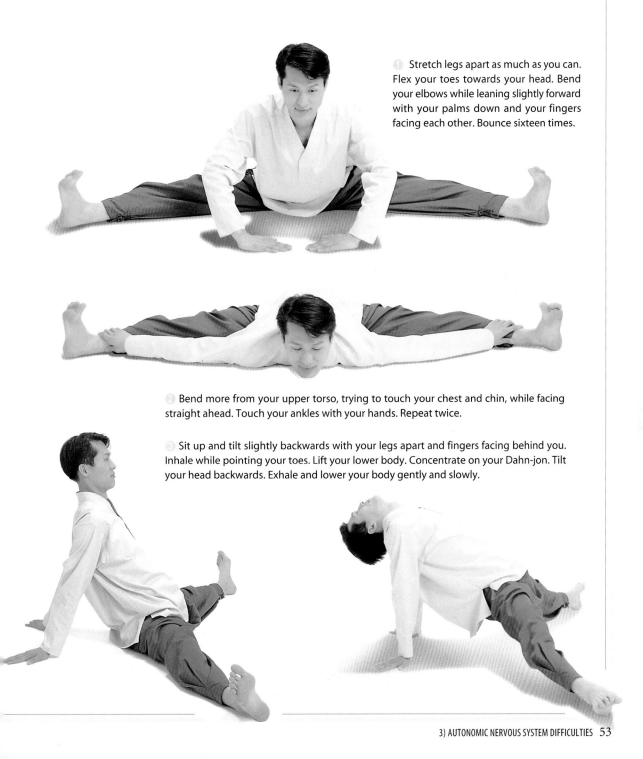

① Stretch legs apart as much as you can. Flex your toes towards your head. Bend your elbows while leaning slightly forward with your palms down and your fingers facing each other. Bounce sixteen times.

② Bend more from your upper torso, trying to touch your chest and chin, while facing straight ahead. Touch your ankles with your hands. Repeat twice.

③ Sit up and tilt slightly backwards with your legs apart and fingers facing behind you. Inhale while pointing your toes. Lift your lower body. Concentrate on your Dahn-jon. Tilt your head backwards. Exhale and lower your body gently and slowly.

4) TINGLING/NUMBNESS IN THE HANDS AND FEET

The symptoms of tingling, numbness and/ or pain in the hands or feet arise from blockages of the somatic nervous system division of the peripheral nervous system. The blockage occurs in the transmission of peripheral nerve fiber conduction of sensory data or nerve flow to the central nervous system or in blockages of motor nerve fibers extending out to skeletal muscle.

Sometimes, the tingling, numbness, and pain have their etiology in the central nervous system, as when a disease is present in the brain or the spinal bone marrow. Usually however, manifestations of these symptoms are related to peripheral nervous system blockages.

When a person experiences a cardio-vascular accident (CVA/Stroke) in the brain, symptoms occurring in one hemisphere of the brain will adversely affect the feet and hands of the opposite side of the body from the hemisphere of the brain which was affected by the stroke.

If you practice the exercises that follow, you can access and utilize Ki energy to innervate the flow and circulation of blood, thereby nourishing your muscles and extremities. In addition, you can release stagnant or toxic energy that has accumulated in the peripheral nervous system areas. This will result in attenuation of your symptoms

BODY TAPPING (p. 22)

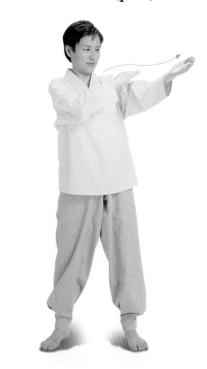

CIRCULATION EXERCISE (p. 26)

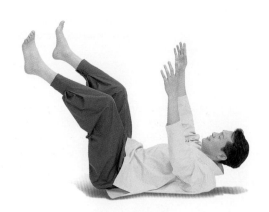

1. ARM SWINGS

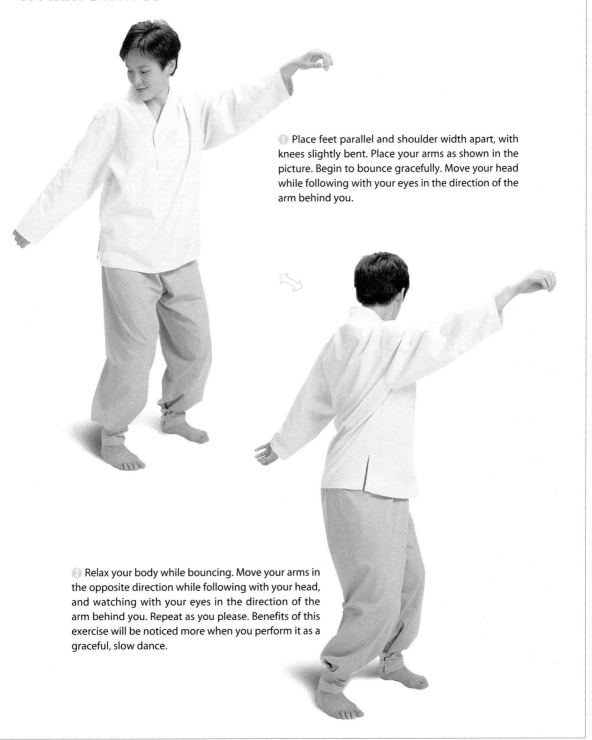

● Place feet parallel and shoulder width apart, with knees slightly bent. Place your arms as shown in the picture. Begin to bounce gracefully. Move your head while following with your eyes in the direction of the arm behind you.

● Relax your body while bouncing. Move your arms in the opposite direction while following with your head, and watching with your eyes in the direction of the arm behind you. Repeat as you please. Benefits of this exercise will be noticed more when you perform it as a graceful, slow dance.

2. SUPERMAN POSTURE

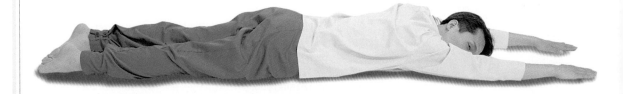

① Lie on your stomach with your arms extended as shown in the picture.

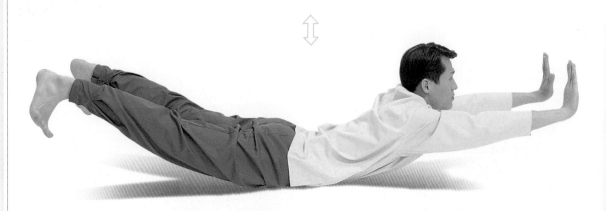

② Inhale. Lift your head up. Look straight ahead. Lift your hands and feet. Make a 90-degree angle with your wrists and feet. With advanced practice, you can employ Dahn-jon breathing to enhance the benefits of this exercise.

③ Exhale. Return to STEP 1.

3. BOAT POSTURE

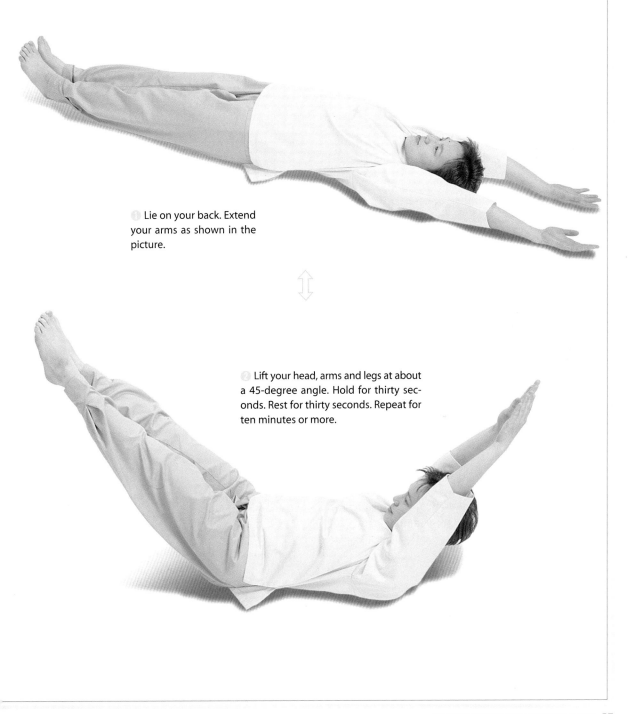

① Lie on your back. Extend your arms as shown in the picture.

② Lift your head, arms and legs at about a 45-degree angle. Hold for thirty seconds. Rest for thirty seconds. Repeat for ten minutes or more.

2. ENDOCRINE SYSTEM

1) THYROID DISORDERS

❧

The Thyroid gland produces thyroid hormones. In addition, when the baby is in the uterus, the thyroid gland, which is shaped like a bow tie, moves from its upper neck location, to a more central neck location just before birth. Somehow, in a number of cases, it does not quite descend to the more centrally located position in the neck. We call this condition hyperthyroidism. The excessive production and synthesis of thyroid hormones cause this. In addition, Iodine, which comes from the water we drink and the food we eat, becomes concentrated in excess in the thyroid gland. Symptoms can include: sweating, weight loss due to increased basal metabolism, palpitations, nervousness, fatigue, hypersensitivity to heat, insomnia, GI disturbances in the form of frequent bowel movements, and other imbalances in the regulation of the autonomic nervous system. In severe cases, one can develop goiter. Graves disease is often diagnosed in the case of hyperthyroidism.

The following exercises will help to restore balance in thyroid functioning. If you have an under-activity of thyroid functioning, known as hypothyroidism, these exercises will be beneficial as well.

1. EXPANDING THE CHEST AND PUSHING THE ARMS

TIPS When you push your arms out, hold the wrists at a 90-degree angle. Turn your head and follow with your eyes to the arm behind you. When you turn your head, you should feel tension in the opposite side of the neck from which your head is facing.

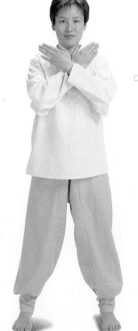

① Place your feet parallel and shoulder width apart. Cross your arms in front of your chest, with your palms facing your chest.

CIRCULATION EXERCISE (p. 26)

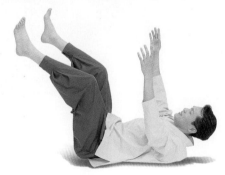

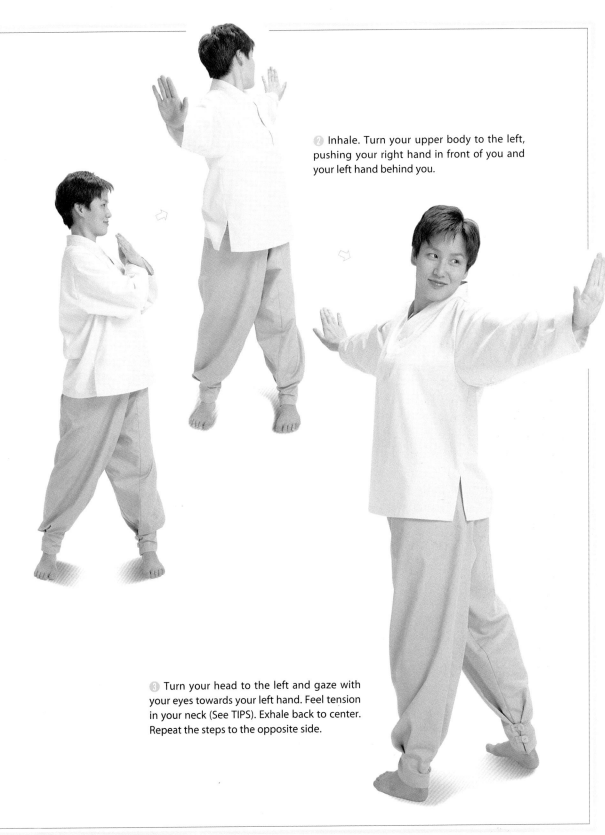

2 Inhale. Turn your upper body to the left, pushing your right hand in front of you and your left hand behind you.

3 Turn your head to the left and gaze with your eyes towards your left hand. Feel tension in your neck (See TIPS). Exhale back to center. Repeat the steps to the opposite side.

2. STANDING FORWARD BEND

Benefits This exercise stimulates the Urinary Bladder Meridian and enhances balanced thyroid functioning. The Dok-maek is energized. This enhances proficiency of blood circulation to the heart. It optimizes functioning of the arm and shoulder muscles, liver, and other organs.

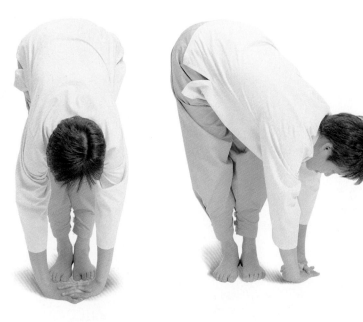

① Place your feet together. Lock your fingers. Inhale as you bend your upper body from your trunk, as you begin to bounce gently. Keep your knees straight, but not tensed. Try to touch your palms to the floor in front of you. Then place your palms alternately to either side of your feet.

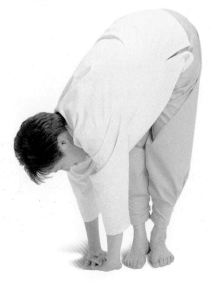

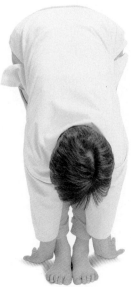

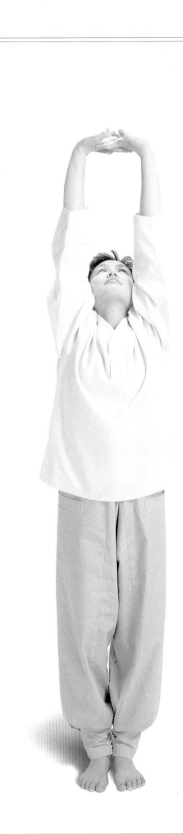

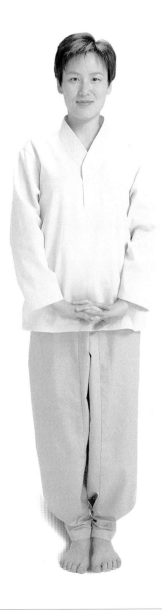

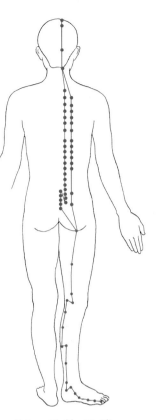

Urinary Bladder Meridian

❷ Raise your upper body to standing with your fingers still locked. Stretch your arms above your head, moving your head back. Follow the stretch and look up at your hands. Exhale and bring your hands down to your Dahn-jon.

3. STRETCHING TOWARD HEAVEN

❶ Place your feet shoulder width apart. Make fists with your hands and bend your arms as shown in the picture.

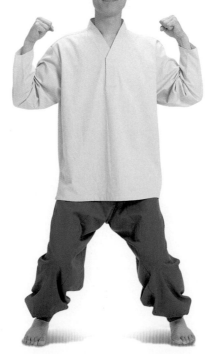

❷ Inhale. Bend your knees. Stretch both arms above your head.

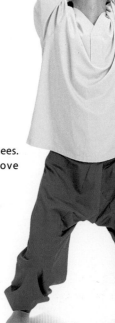

❸ Keep your spine straight as you stretch your fingers up towards the sky. Follow with your eyes to your fingertips. Exhale. Return to STEP 1. Repeat twice.

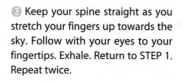

4. HEAD LIFT

Benefits This exercise will help you to accumulate Ki energy through your neck to your brain. This will stimulate the thyroid gland and assist it in the production of thyroid hormone.

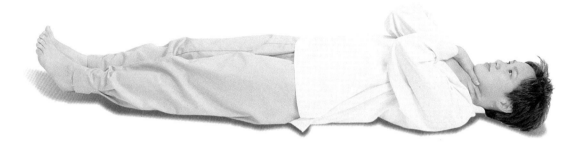

① Lie on your back. Open your thumbs and index fingers of both hands. Place both your hands on the front of your neck as shown in the picture.

⇕

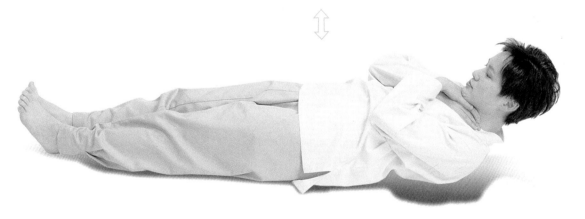

② Inhale. Lift your head with your chin towards your chest. Hold this position for ten seconds, while you gently squeeze your neck with your hands.

③ Exhale through your mouth and return to STEP 1. Repeat one more time.

5. LIFTING LEGS OVER HEAD

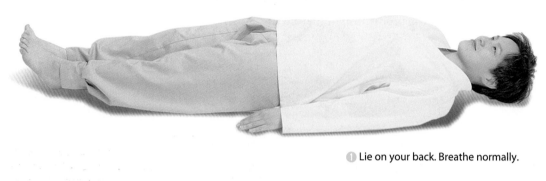

➊ Lie on your back. Breathe normally.

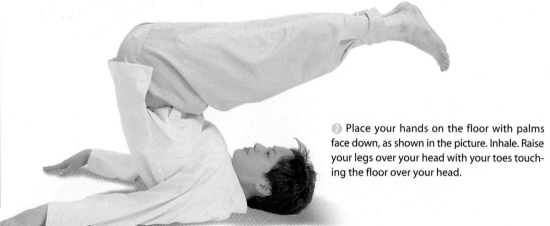

➋ Place your hands on the floor with palms face down, as shown in the picture. Inhale. Raise your legs over your head with your toes touching the floor over your head.

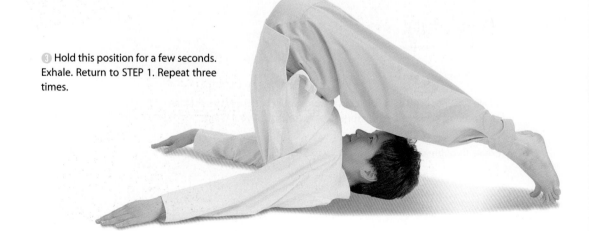

➌ Hold this position for a few seconds. Exhale. Return to STEP 1. Repeat three times.

6. TILTING UPPER BODY BACKWARDS

TIPS   When you tilt your body backwards, touch your heels to your buttocks. The heels and the back of your head face each other during the backward tilt.

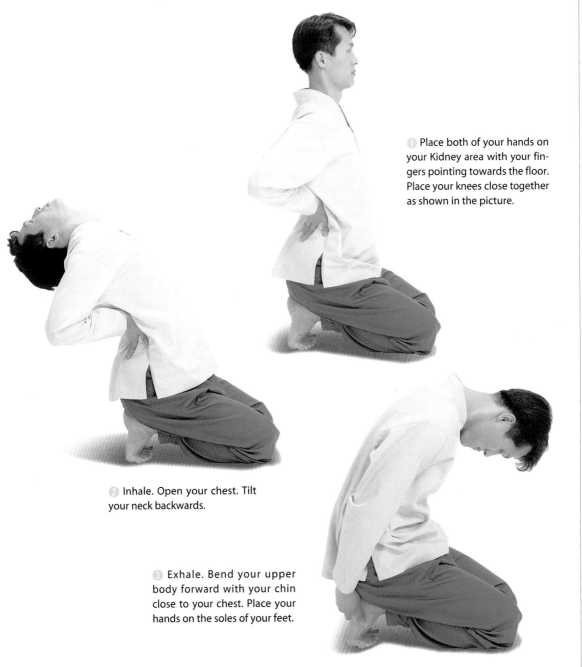

❶ Place both of your hands on your Kidney area with your fingers pointing towards the floor. Place your knees close together as shown in the picture.

❷ Inhale. Open your chest. Tilt your neck backwards.

❸ Exhale. Bend your upper body forward with your chin close to your chest. Place your hands on the soles of your feet.

7. LUNGE WITH HEAD LIFT

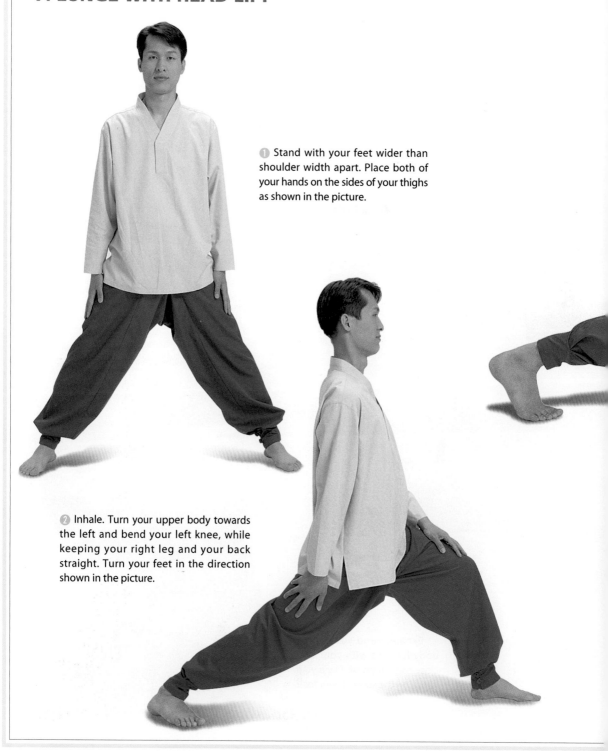

❶ Stand with your feet wider than shoulder width apart. Place both of your hands on the sides of your thighs as shown in the picture.

❷ Inhale. Turn your upper body towards the left and bend your left knee, while keeping your right leg and your back straight. Turn your feet in the direction shown in the picture.

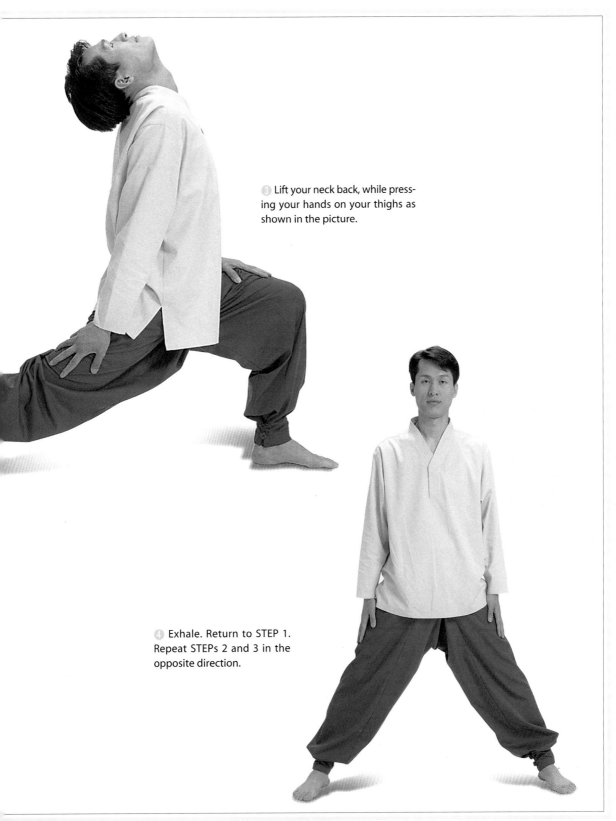

❸ Lift your neck back, while pressing your hands on your thighs as shown in the picture.

❹ Exhale. Return to STEP 1. Repeat STEPs 2 and 3 in the opposite direction.

8. ARM TWIST

You can perform this exercise standing or sitting on your knees.

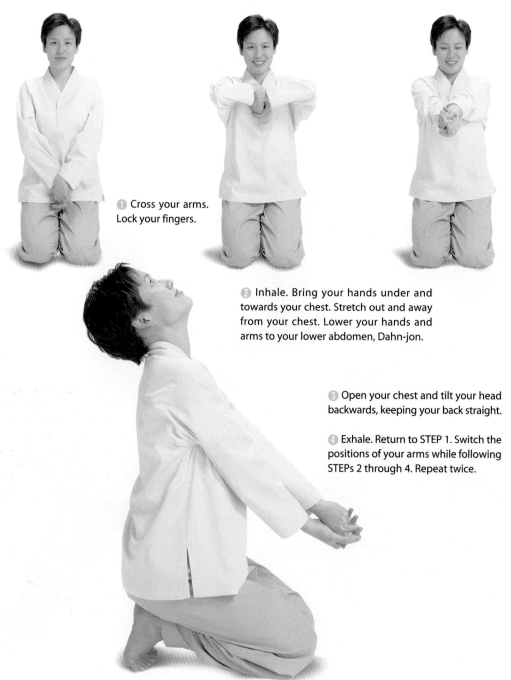

① Cross your arms. Lock your fingers.

② Inhale. Bring your hands under and towards your chest. Stretch out and away from your chest. Lower your hands and arms to your lower abdomen, Dahn-jon.

③ Open your chest and tilt your head backwards, keeping your back straight.

④ Exhale. Return to STEP 1. Switch the positions of your arms while following STEPs 2 through 4. Repeat twice.

9. NECK TILTING BACKWARD WITH BACK TEETH TOUCHING

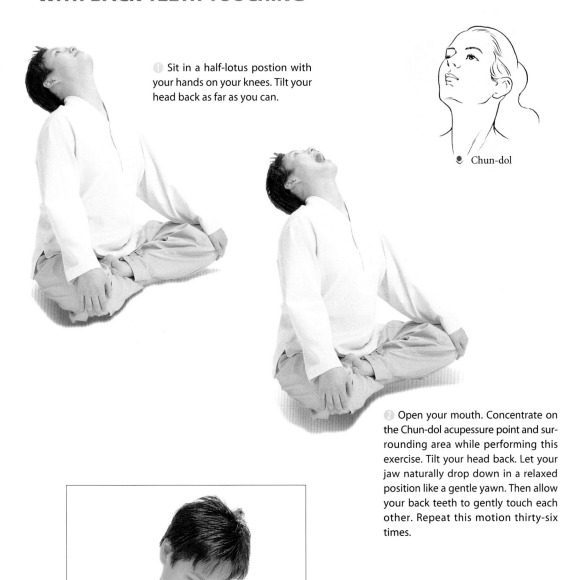

① Sit in a half-lotus postion with your hands on your knees. Tilt your head back as far as you can.

Chun-dol

② Open your mouth. Concentrate on the Chun-dol acupessure point and surrounding area while performing this exercise. Tilt your head back. Let your jaw naturally drop down in a relaxed position like a gentle yawn. Then allow your back teeth to gently touch each other. Repeat this motion thirty-six times.

③ Rotate your neck very slowly in a circular motion, clockwise and then counter-clockwise to relax your neck muscles.

2) DIABETES

Diabetes is a term that refers several disorders diagnosed when there is excessive urine being excreted by the individual. It is believed that the pancreas cannot create enough insulin or the increased production of insulin is not effective. diabetes insipidus (known as "water diabetes,") arises when there is a deficiency of anti-diuretic hormone due to a dysfunction of the pituitary gland and/or kidney.

The dominant precursors of diabetes are genetic predisposition, environmental factors, obesity, or age factors. In addition, mental stress is thought to be a significant etiological factor in the development of this disease. Treatment includes diet, self-monitoring of blood sugar, compliance with any prescribed medication, and exercise.

Exercise performed daily and consistently is imperative. It is important to develop self-management skills in regulating diabetes in the areas discussed above. Dahnhak exercises that are recommended in this book are based on the self-management principle. Dahn-jon breathing, which is a holistic meditative form of respiration, boosts the immune system, and allows the blood to circulate, enabling more stable insulin regulation by the pancreas. Through these Dahnhak exercises, alpha waves are accessed. This results in the promotion of a sense of serenity experienced in mind and body, as brain function is enhanced. This is enormously helpful for diabetics, as they have a tendency for elevated levels of tension.

TOE TAPPING (p. 34)

Benefits helps to bring fire energy down to the Dahn-jon

JOK-SAM-NI HITTING (p. 38)

Benefits Stimulates the Stomach Meridian and relieves stagnant energy.

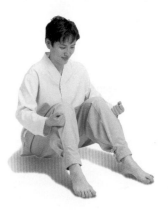

UPPER BODY LIFT (p. 50)

Benefits Stimulates insulin secretion and aligns spinal cord and enhances kidney, bladder, and reproductive system.

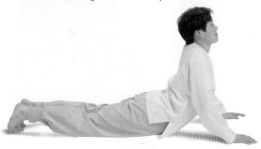

1. RAISING HANDS

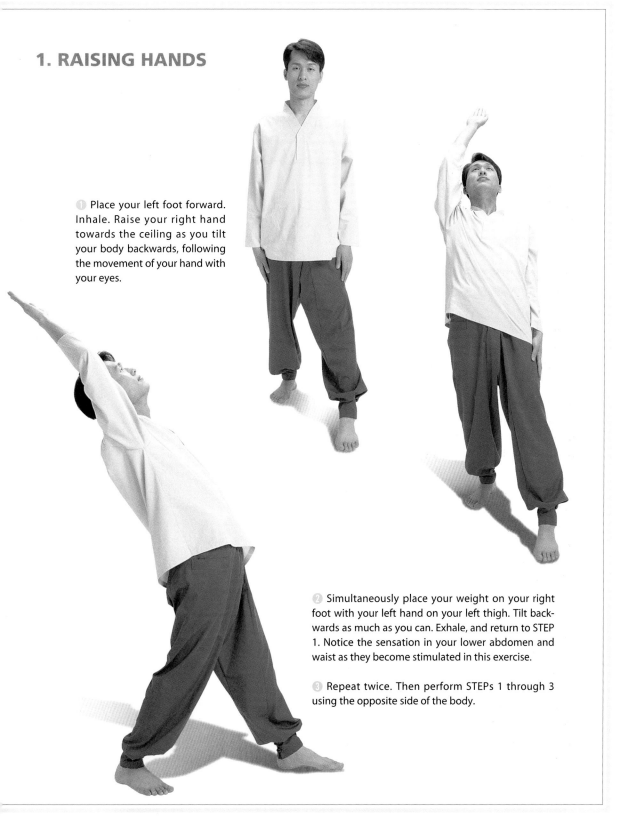

① Place your left foot forward. Inhale. Raise your right hand towards the ceiling as you tilt your body backwards, following the movement of your hand with your eyes.

② Simultaneously place your weight on your right foot with your left hand on your left thigh. Tilt backwards as much as you can. Exhale, and return to STEP 1. Notice the sensation in your lower abdomen and waist as they become stimulated in this exercise.

③ Repeat twice. Then perform STEPs 1 through 3 using the opposite side of the body.

2. ROTATING PLATE

Benefits Enables joint flexibility and mobility. Strengthens autonomic nervous system while enhancing optimal organ function, strengthens immune system and helps to prevent and treat age related problems.

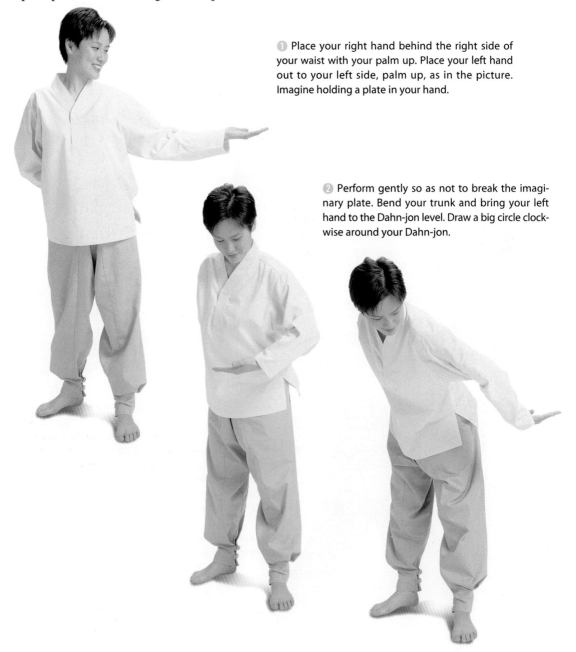

❶ Place your right hand behind the right side of your waist with your palm up. Place your left hand out to your left side, palm up, as in the picture. Imagine holding a plate in your hand.

❷ Perform gently so as not to break the imaginary plate. Bend your trunk and bring your left hand to the Dahn-jon level. Draw a big circle clockwise around your Dahn-jon.

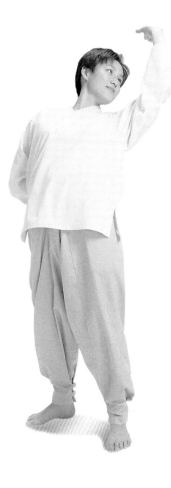

3 Draw an opposite "S" shape towards your head and encircle your head clockwise. Draw an "S" shape as you return, with your left palm up at your left side. Throughout the exercise, concentrate on keeping your plate intact and follow your hand movements with your eyes.

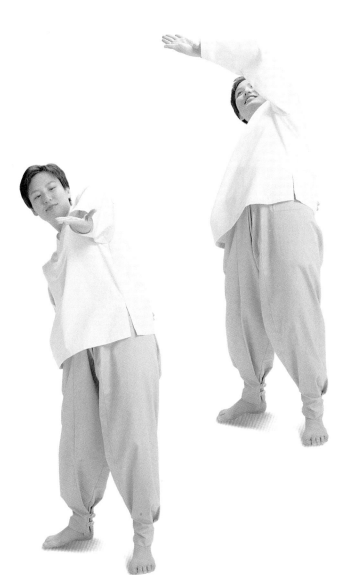

4 Perform the above Steps with your right hand. Alternate your hands while repeating this exercise ten times. Progress to drawing larger circles and "S" shapes with practice.

3. TWISTING AND BENDING THE UPPER BODY WITH LOCKED FINGERS

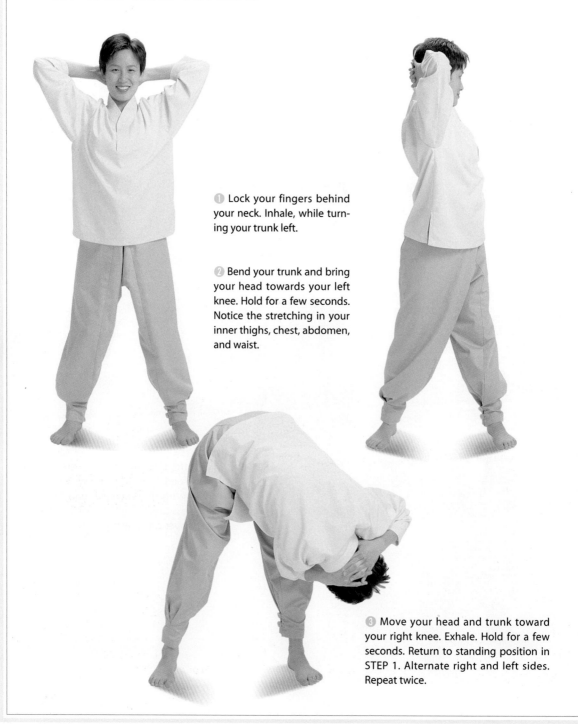

① Lock your fingers behind your neck. Inhale, while turning your trunk left.

② Bend your trunk and bring your head towards your left knee. Hold for a few seconds. Notice the stretching in your inner thighs, chest, abdomen, and waist.

③ Move your head and trunk toward your right knee. Exhale. Hold for a few seconds. Return to standing position in STEP 1. Alternate right and left sides. Repeat twice.

4. GRASPING TOES WHILE PUSHING AND PULLING

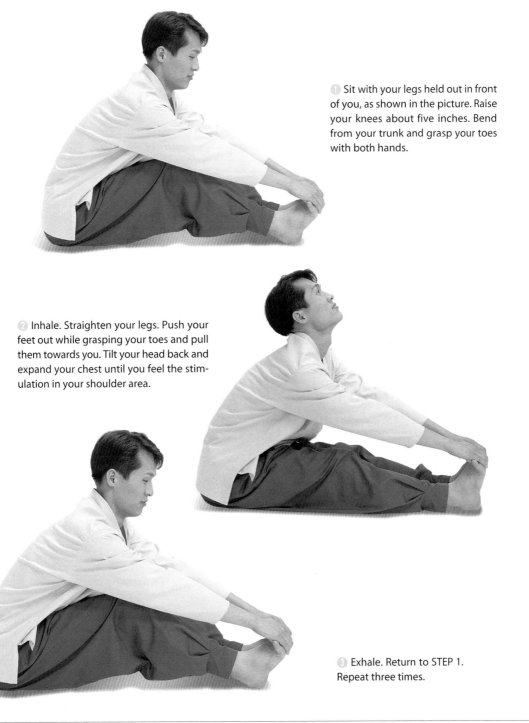

① Sit with your legs held out in front of you, as shown in the picture. Raise your knees about five inches. Bend from your trunk and grasp your toes with both hands.

② Inhale. Straighten your legs. Push your feet out while grasping your toes and pull them towards you. Tilt your head back and expand your chest until you feel the stimulation in your shoulder area.

③ Exhale. Return to STEP 1. Repeat three times.

5. FLAGPOLE POSTURE

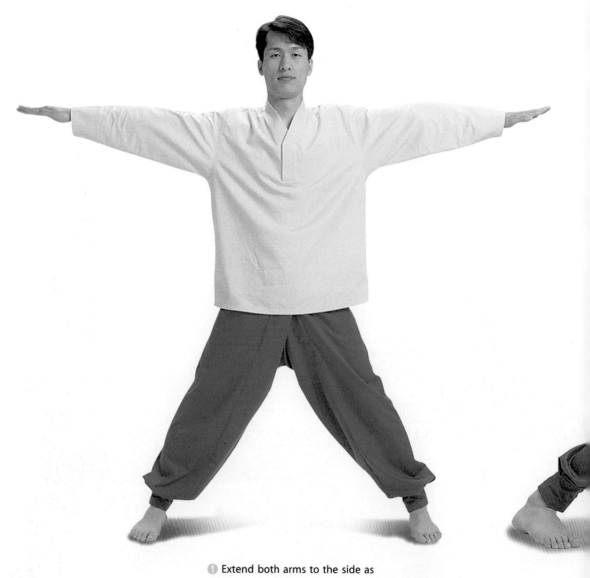

① Extend both arms to the side as shown in the picture. Inhale. Turn your trunk to the left.

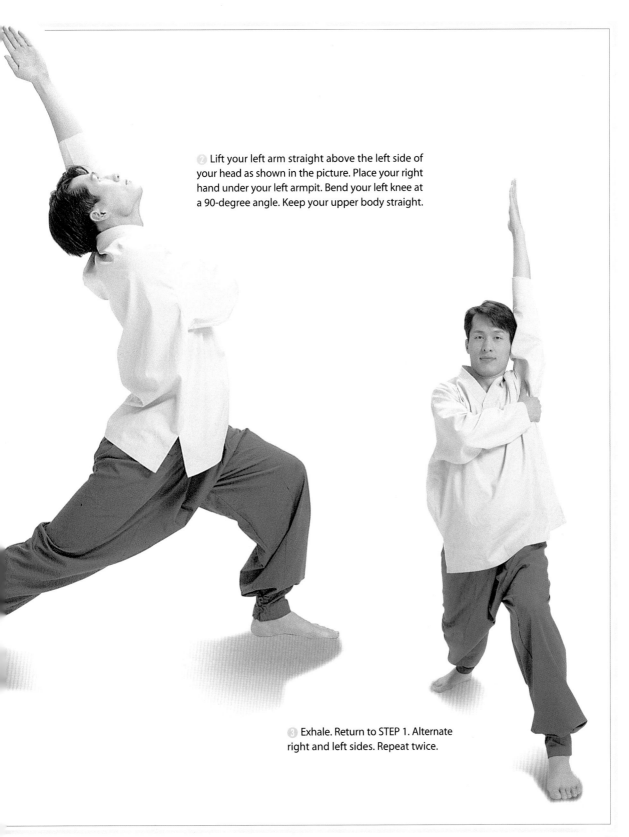

❷ Lift your left arm straight above the left side of your head as shown in the picture. Place your right hand under your left armpit. Bend your left knee at a 90-degree angle. Keep your upper body straight.

❸ Exhale. Return to STEP 1. Alternate right and left sides. Repeat twice.

6. TURNING FEET IN

Benefits It strengthens the lower Dahn-jon and lower extremities, and stimulates the Spleen Meridian. As you progress in the practice of this Hang-gong exercise, you will be able to more readily detect the flow of energy through the Spleen Meridian, beginning at the feet and moving up to the spleen.

TIPS Do not stiffen the muscles above the navel where your spleen and pancreas are located.

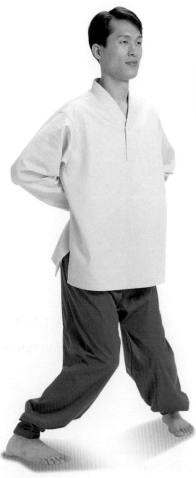

❶ Stand with legs shoulder width apart, with your toes at a 45-degree angle, pointing inwards. Your knees are almost touching, and your spine is straight.

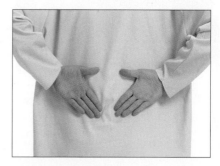

❷ Place both hands behind you where your Kidneys are located, with your palms turned outward, as shown in the picture.

❸ In this posture, you can notice your Dahn-jon area become taut. Perform this posture for five minutes in the beginning. As you progress in practice, perform for thirty to forty minutes.

7. CROSSING LEGS AND TWISTING

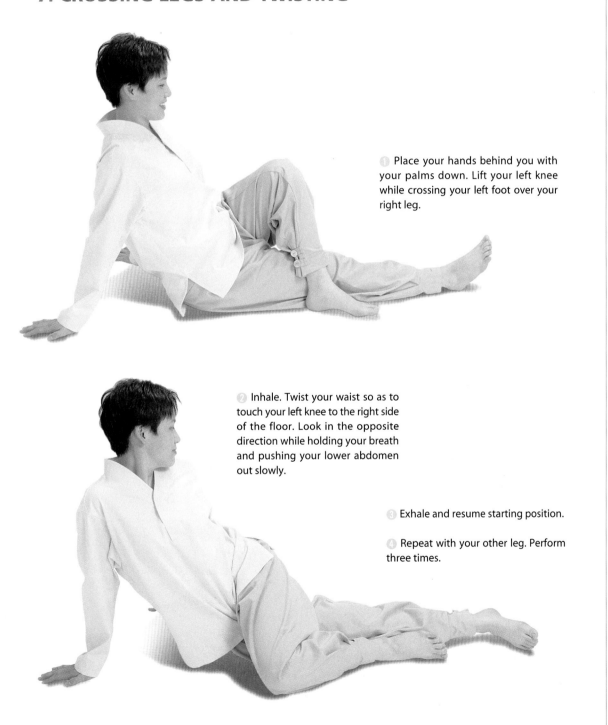

① Place your hands behind you with your palms down. Lift your left knee while crossing your left foot over your right leg.

② Inhale. Twist your waist so as to touch your left knee to the right side of the floor. Look in the opposite direction while holding your breath and pushing your lower abdomen out slowly.

③ Exhale and resume starting position.

④ Repeat with your other leg. Perform three times.

3. RESPIRATORY SYSTEM

1) LUNG DISEASE

The primary purpose of the respiratory system is to provide oxygen to the body, while ridding the system of carbon dioxide and toxic inhalants. This is accomplished through a complex series of communications and events between several key areas of the body including the respiratory center of the brain, the chest wall, the musculoskeletal system, the nervous system, and, of course, the lungs.

Lung disease can be caused by environmental factors such as smoking and other air pollutants. The Lung Meridian is related to intense emotions. If, for example, you are very sad or grieving, the lungs can become impaired. Conditions of sadness or grieving can cause compression of the chest, and diminished capacity of proper breathing, which can lead to disease. Through Dahn-jon breathing, pressure is decreased in the lungs, enabling the chest to expand, the rib cage to be properly placed, and symmetry and spinal alignment to be achieved. Proficient breathing is thereby established, and circulation of oxygen and the releasing of carbon dioxide and other toxins from the body is expedited. As you perform the following Dahnhak exercises described in this section, you will notice an overall heightened sense of well-being, as your respiratory system becomes more resilient. The increase in the flow of oxygen will result in increased energy and concentrated focus. This will reverberate throughout your body and enable your search for your overall mind/body/spirit self-healing mission.

STRETCHING TOWARD HEAVEN (p. 62)

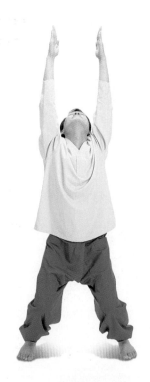

MOVING A JAR (p. 49)

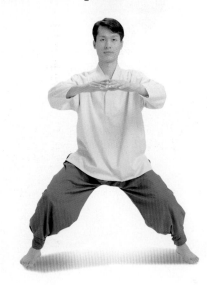

1. CLASPED HANDS FORWARD BEND

Benefits Expands chest to enhance and strengthen blood circulation in the lungs and endocrine system. Facilitates more rapid transit time for elimination.

TIPS Keep spine lengthened, not rigid. If lotus position is too difficult, then you can perform in a half-lotus postion or with legs crossed.

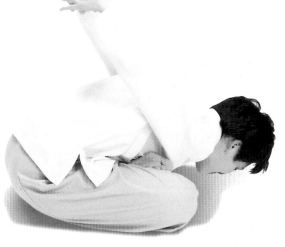

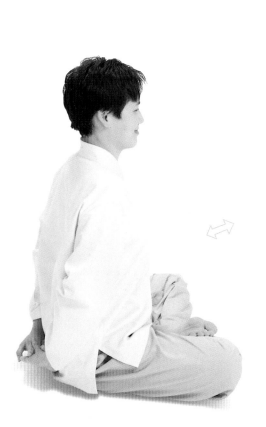

❷ While keeping spine lengthened yet not rigid, bend your upper body from the trunk. Simultaneously lift both arms towards the back of your head.

❸ Return to STEP 1. Repeat three times.

❶ Sit in a half-lotus postion. Lock your fingers behind you

2. CLAPSED HANDS STRETCH AND BEND

Benefits This stretch allows the spine, rib cage, and organs to achieve proper alignment to enhance the function of the respiratory system. As you stretch up towards the sky, stagnant energy is released from the shoulders and under the arms (where lymph glands are located). This ameliorates stomach distress. As you stretch towards the floor, flexibility of your neck, spine, and waist is achieved.

TIPS When you push with both arms above your head towards the sky, follow this movement with your eyes. However, if dizziness occurs, or you have a history of anemia or hypertension, then fix your eyes straight ahead in executing this movement. Do not force this stretch. Rather, proceed with a gentle challenge.

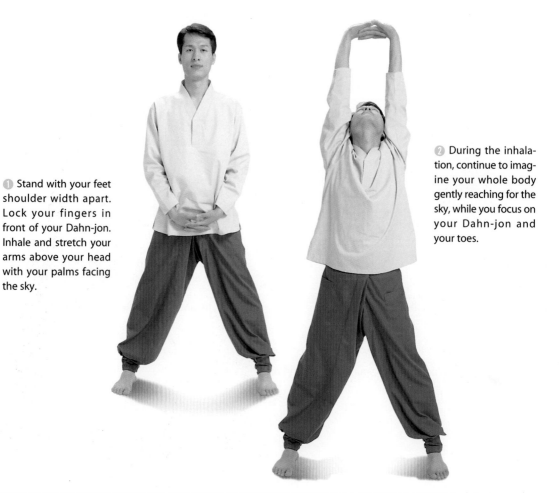

① Stand with your feet shoulder width apart. Lock your fingers in front of your Dahn-jon. Inhale and stretch your arms above your head with your palms facing the sky.

② During the inhalation, continue to imagine your whole body gently reaching for the sky, while you focus on your Dahn-jon and your toes.

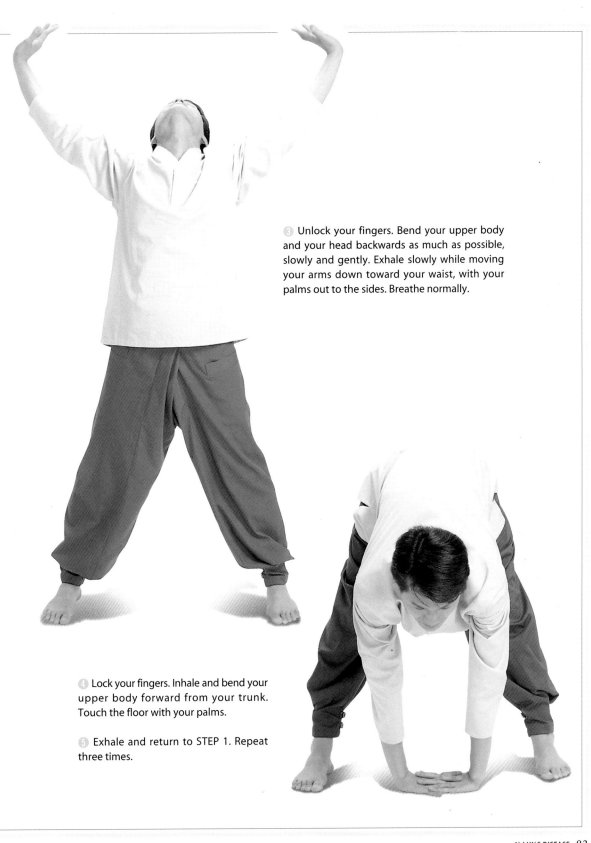

❸ Unlock your fingers. Bend your upper body and your head backwards as much as possible, slowly and gently. Exhale slowly while moving your arms down toward your waist, with your palms out to the sides. Breathe normally.

❹ Lock your fingers. Inhale and bend your upper body forward from your trunk. Touch the floor with your palms.

❺ Exhale and return to STEP 1. Repeat three times.

3. SWEEPING DOWN CHEST WITH HANDS

Benefits Releases stagnant energy in the lungs and enhances blood circulation

Place both hands on your chest as shown in the picture. Sweep your chest with downward strokes while simultaneously focusing your attention on your inhalation and exhalation, which should be executed slowly, deeply, and gently.

4. WRIST SHAKING

Benefits When you shake your wrists, stagnant energy is released from the Lung Meridian to augment strengthening of the lungs and other organs.

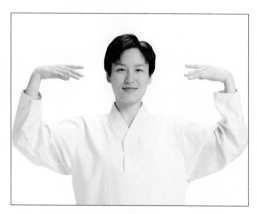

Open your chest. Hold arms as shown in the picture. Shake your wrists.

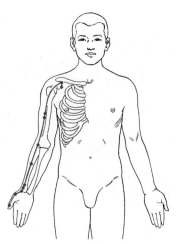

Lung Meridian
(extends from thumb to lung)

5. HANG-GONG FOR STRENGTHENING THE LUNGS

Benefits Strengthens spinal cord and lungs and innervates the accumulation of fire energy of the lungs. Expedites recovery from lung problems.

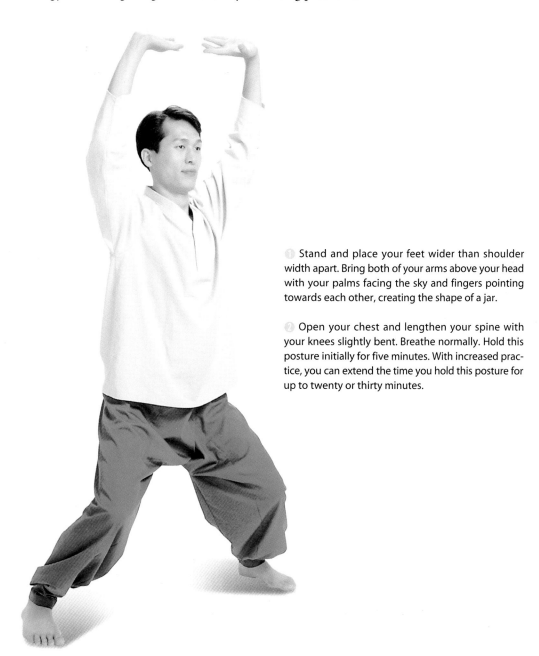

1 Stand and place your feet wider than shoulder width apart. Bring both of your arms above your head with your palms facing the sky and fingers pointing towards each other, creating the shape of a jar.

2 Open your chest and lengthen your spine with your knees slightly bent. Breathe normally. Hold this posture initially for five minutes. With increased practice, you can extend the time you hold this posture for up to twenty or thirty minutes.

6. CHEST EXPANSION

Benefits Strengthens the heart and the lungs. Releases Fire Energy. Decreases symptoms of blushing and/or hot flashes.

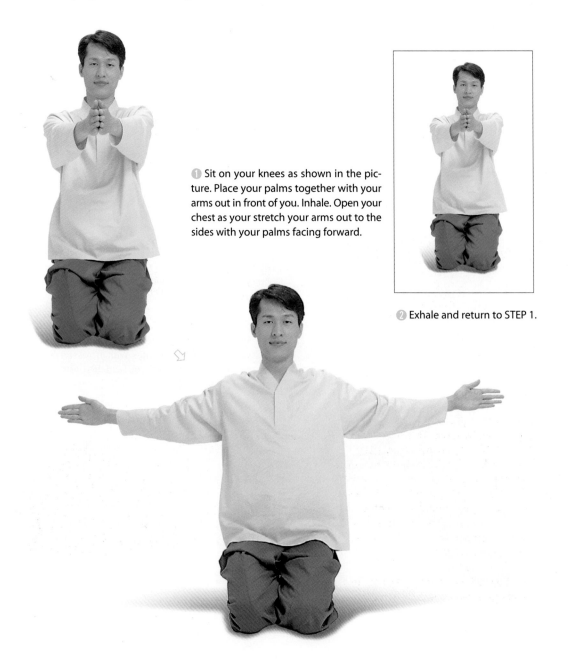

❶ Sit on your knees as shown in the picture. Place your palms together with your arms out in front of you. Inhale. Open your chest as your stretch your arms out to the sides with your palms facing forward.

❷ Exhale and return to STEP 1.

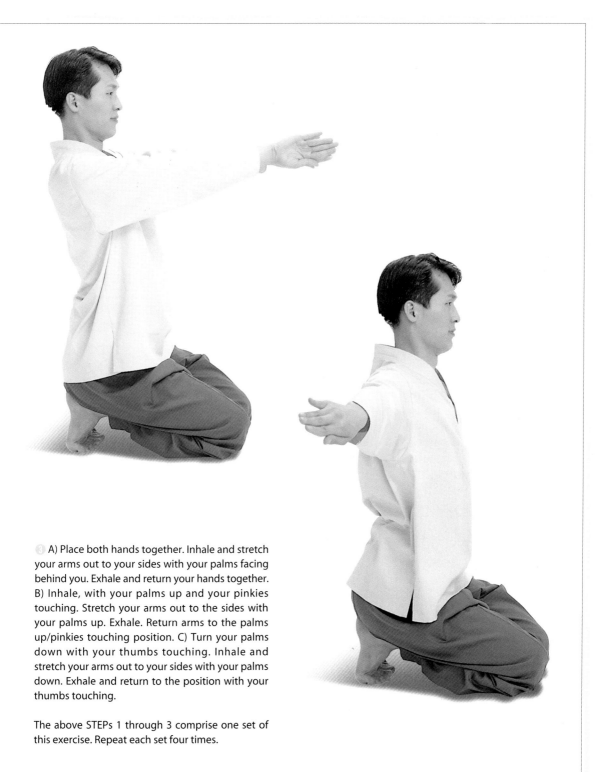

A) Place both hands together. Inhale and stretch your arms out to your sides with your palms facing behind you. Exhale and return your hands together. B) Inhale, with your palms up and your pinkies touching. Stretch your arms out to the sides with your palms up. Exhale. Return arms to the palms up/pinkies touching position. C) Turn your palms down with your thumbs touching. Inhale and stretch your arms out to your sides with your palms down. Exhale and return to the position with your thumbs touching.

The above STEPs 1 through 3 comprise one set of this exercise. Repeat each set four times.

7. ROTATING THE SHOULDERS

Benefits Relaxes the shoulders and facilitates blood circulation. Expands the chest to allow for symmetry and alignment of the spine and organs so they can function at their maximum capacity.

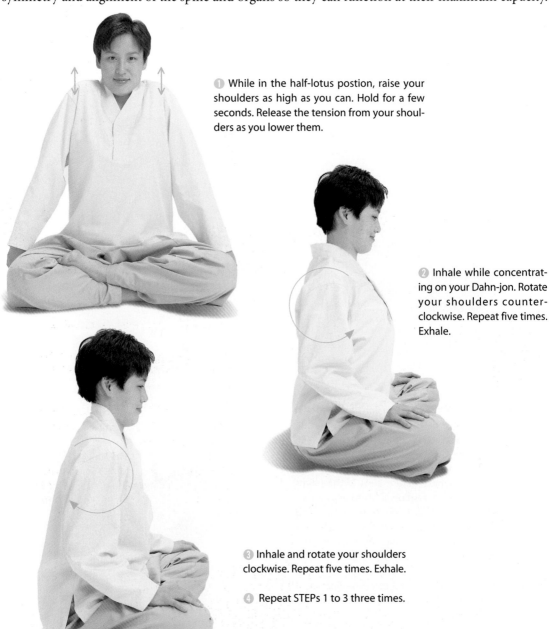

❶ While in the half-lotus postion, raise your shoulders as high as you can. Hold for a few seconds. Release the tension from your shoulders as you lower them.

❷ Inhale while concentrating on your Dahn-jon. Rotate your shoulders counterclockwise. Repeat five times. Exhale.

❸ Inhale and rotate your shoulders clockwise. Repeat five times. Exhale.

❹ Repeat STEPs 1 to 3 three times.

8. PULLING KNEE TOWARD THE CHEST

Benefits Facilitates blood and lung circulation. Aligns the cervical spine.

TIPS When you pull your knee towards your chest, inhale, open your chest, and exert gentle tension with your arms, shoulders, waist and Dahn-jon. Simultaneously flex your opposite foot, so toes are pointing towards you.

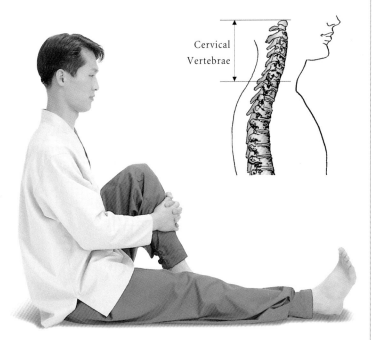

Cervical Vertebrae

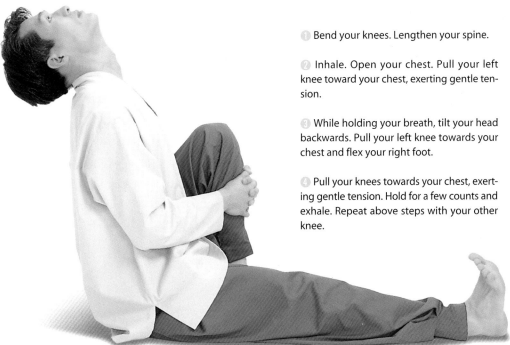

❶ Bend your knees. Lengthen your spine.

❷ Inhale. Open your chest. Pull your left knee toward your chest, exerting gentle tension.

❸ While holding your breath, tilt your head backwards. Pull your left knee towards your chest and flex your right foot.

❹ Pull your knees towards your chest, exerting gentle tension. Hold for a few counts and exhale. Repeat above steps with your other knee.

3. RESPIRATORY SYSTEM

2) COLD/FLU

∽೧

When you practice Dahnhak exercise consistently, the immune system is boosted, thus thwarting the onset of colds and the flu. If the system is compromised and one does come down with a cold or the flu, the symptoms will be milder, and recovery will be faster. Proponents of Western Medicine believe that colds/flu are caused by viruses. Eastern Medicine adherents believe that when the conditions in the environment are cold, moist and damp, the energy produced by these factors enters the body system. Treatment consists of releasing the cold energy from the body.

The cold, damp, moist energy will initally enter through the back of the neck called the "Poong-moon" acupressure point. It is imperative, particularly during the change of season, to ensure that warmth is maintained in these areas. Early symptoms signaling the onset of a cold is the experiencing of chills and a runny nose.

Dahnhak Meridian exercises stimulate the body to enhance the flow of Ki energy, boost the immune system, and thwart the onset or decrease the severity of colds/flu. Colds are not serious, but if prolonged, pneumonia, tuberculosis, or heart disease can develop.

CLASPED HANDS FORWARD BEND (p. 81)

Benefits Assists in recovery from colds, cough, bronchitis, emphysema, and difficulty breathing. After this exercise, tilt your head back. Open your mouth and concentrate on the Chun-dol acupressure point. Let your jaw drop naturally. Allow your back teeth to gently touch each other. Repeat thirty-six times. See page 69- Neck Tilting Backward With Back Teeth Touching.

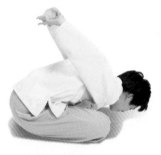

TO PREVENT COLDS

Benefits Helps clear congestion from colds. Prevents or lessens duration of cold.

Method Perform this exercise upon awakening in the morning. Inhale. Using both middle fingers, rub them against each other to create heat energy. Then breathe naturally while you place your fingers on the Dae-chu acuressure points and press and massage for about five minutes.

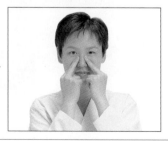

1. STRENGTHENING TOES

Benefits Boosts metabolism and immune system, burns fat cells in upper and lower body, and enhances blood and energy circulation.

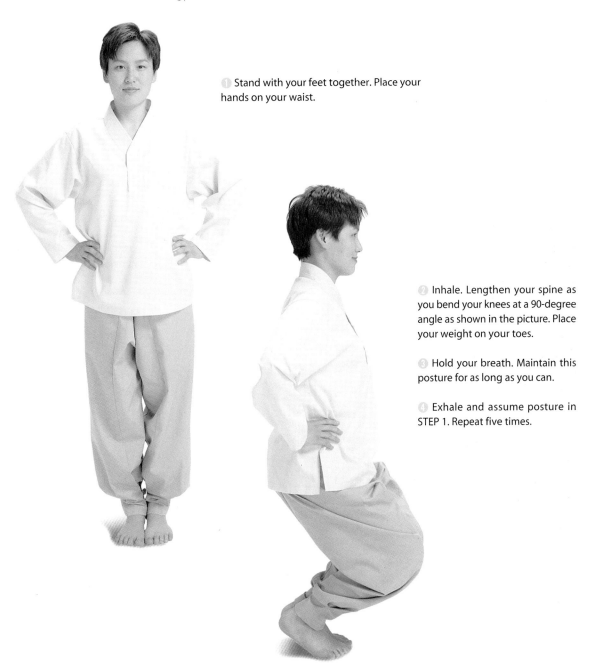

1 Stand with your feet together. Place your hands on your waist.

2 Inhale. Lengthen your spine as you bend your knees at a 90-degree angle as shown in the picture. Place your weight on your toes.

3 Hold your breath. Maintain this posture for as long as you can.

4 Exhale and assume posture in STEP 1. Repeat five times.

2. SHOULDER STRETCHING

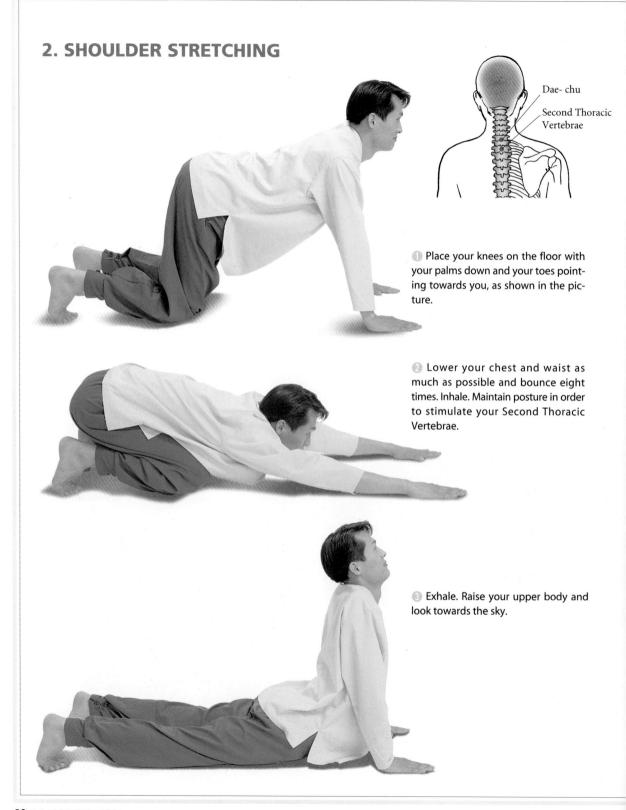

Dae- chu

Second Thoracic
Vertebrae

❶ Place your knees on the floor with your palms down and your toes pointing towards you, as shown in the picture.

❷ Lower your chest and waist as much as possible and bounce eight times. Inhale. Maintain posture in order to stimulate your Second Thoracic Vertebrae.

❸ Exhale. Raise your upper body and look towards the sky.

3. DROPPING LIKE A LEAF FROM A TREE

TIPS When you inhale and raise your heels, create tension in your body.
When you exhale, realease all tension.

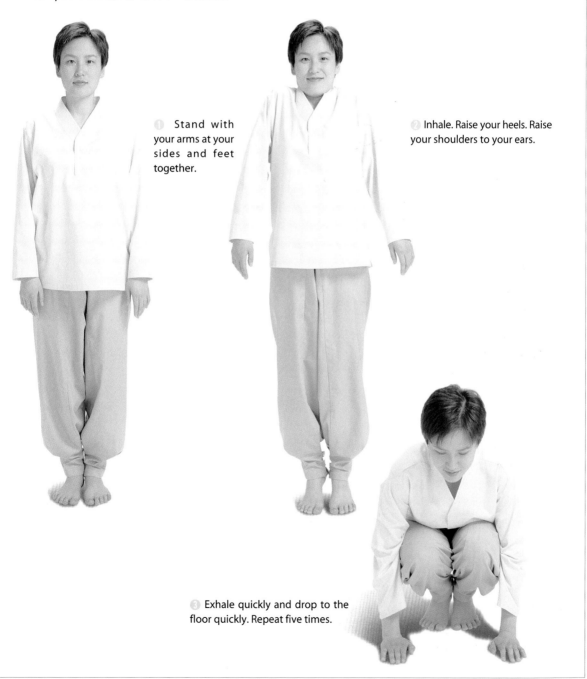

① Stand with your arms at your sides and feet together.

② Inhale. Raise your heels. Raise your shoulders to your ears.

③ Exhale quickly and drop to the floor quickly. Repeat five times.

4. ROWING A BOAT

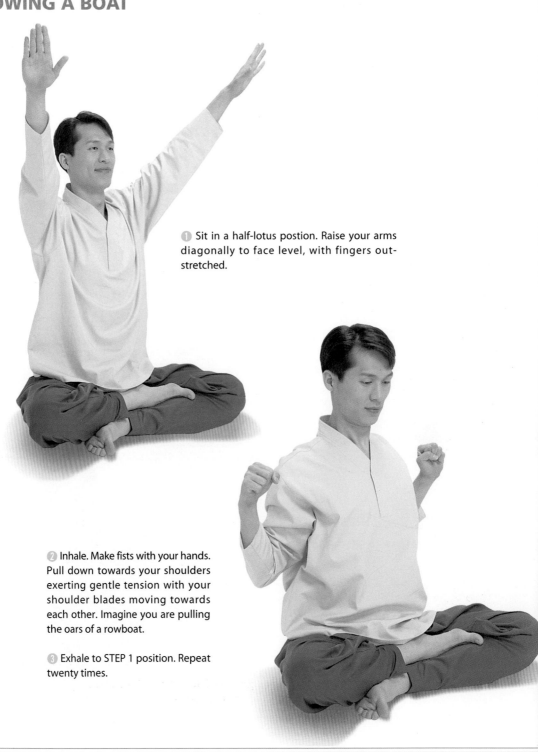

① Sit in a half-lotus postion. Raise your arms diagonally to face level, with fingers outstretched.

② Inhale. Make fists with your hands. Pull down towards your shoulders exerting gentle tension with your shoulder blades moving towards each other. Imagine you are pulling the oars of a rowboat.

③ Exhale to STEP 1 position. Repeat twenty times.

5. HEAD TURNING

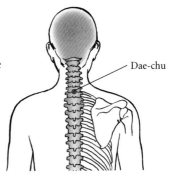

Dae-chu

Benefits Regulates the smooth flow of Ki energy to enable the release of cold energy from the Dae-chu acupressure point.

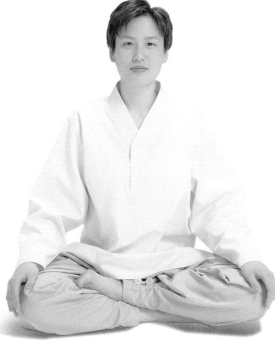

① Sit in a half-lotus position. Lengthen your spine. Place your hands on your knees.

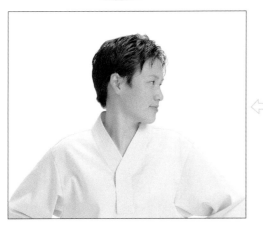 ⟺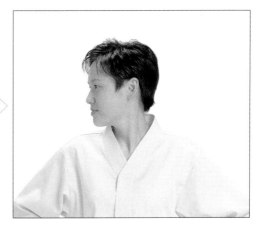

② Slowly turn your head to the right and left thirty times. Concentrate on the Dae-chu point while performing this exercise.

6. SHOULDERSTAND WITH WAIST SUPPORT

Benefits Maximizes Ki energy flow through the neck and brain which helps regulate the thyroid and relieve headaches. Assists in lowering cholesterol, enhancing blood circulation, and detoxifying the blood throughout the body.

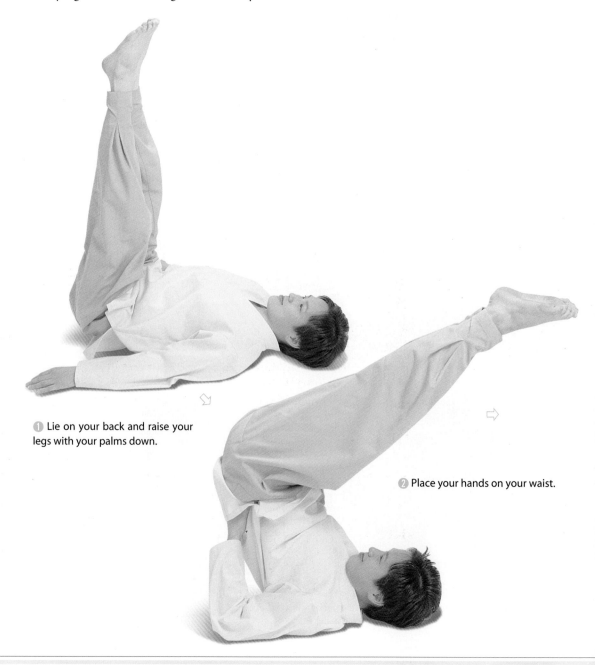

1 Lie on your back and raise your legs with your palms down.

2 Place your hands on your waist.

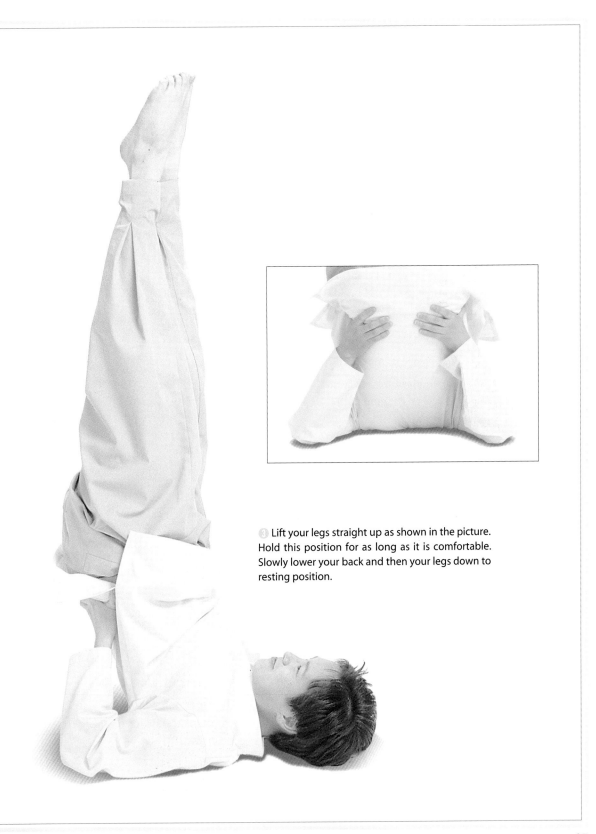

❸ Lift your legs straight up as shown in the picture. Hold this position for as long as it is comfortable. Slowly lower your back and then your legs down to resting position.

4. BONE, MUSCLE, AND SKIN

1) LUMBAGO

Lower back pain is a common malady. The etiology is multifaceted and may include faulty postural habits, sudden, jerky movements, lifting heavy objects improperly, fatigue, deficient or poor quality sleep, and lack of exercise. Tension in the muscles that are located alongside the spine causes them to constrict, which is accompanied by oxygen deprivation.

Tight hamstring muscles adversely affect the pelvis, thereby compromising the lower back, creating tension in muscles and tendons in the lower back. This, in turn, ultimately affects misalignment of the spine, which, in some cases, results in disc damage.

In order to thrive, muscles need purified oxygen transported throughout the blood, so that the impulses in the nerves will activate correctly. By performing Meridian exercises persistently, the muscles will loosen and allow rich, oxygenated blood to flow in an unobstructed fashion into the muscles, nourishing them and permitting energy to circulate throughout the system. Dahnhak practice combines the necessary therapeutic elements of massaging acupressure points and meridians, to maximize efficient energy and blood transportation throughout the body. Relax your body to release tension. Then, very slowly begin to engage the Meridian exercises recommended in this chapter, being mindful of performing only those which can be executed comfortably. It is best not to remain sedentary when afflicted with lumbago, because Ki energy can become obstructed, thus escalating the sensation and perception of pain and stiffness.

INTESTINAL EXERCISE (p. 28)

Benefits This exercise increases heat energy in the Dahn-jon area, which permeates the body, including the lower back, spine, and organs.

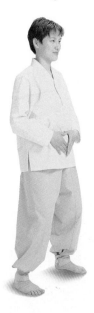

DAHN-JON TAPPING (p. 27)

Benefits This exercise accumulates Ki energy and blood circulation in your Dahn-jon. It also strengthens the lower abdomen and waist area.

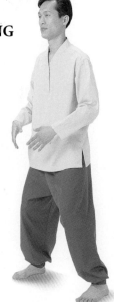

1. SWEEPING DOWN THE BLADDER MERIDIAN

Benefits This exercise increases heat energy in the Dahn-jon area, which permeates the body, including the lower back, spine, and organs. It helps chronic lumbago and establishes an overall feeling of well-being.

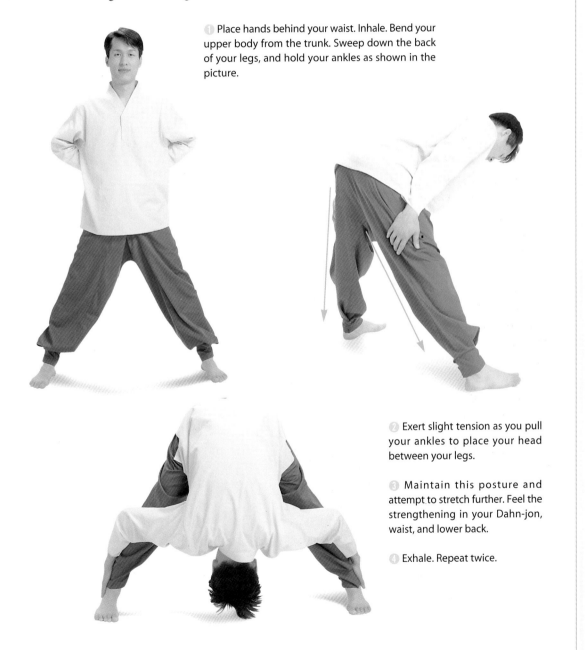

❶ Place hands behind your waist. Inhale. Bend your upper body from the trunk. Sweep down the back of your legs, and hold your ankles as shown in the picture.

❷ Exert slight tension as you pull your ankles to place your head between your legs.

❸ Maintain this posture and attempt to stretch further. Feel the strengthening in your Dahn-jon, waist, and lower back.

❹ Exhale. Repeat twice.

2. LYING HIP BOUNCE

Benefits This exercise opens the Myung-moon acupressure point, allowing the transmission of energy to circulate in the hips and waist. The vibration of the organs from this exercise enables them to become stronger. It also opens the meridians for the lower extremities, enabling efficient energy and blood circulation, and opens up blockages in the waist area. It is an easy exercise to perform.

TIPS Relax your waist and lower extremities while performing this exercise.

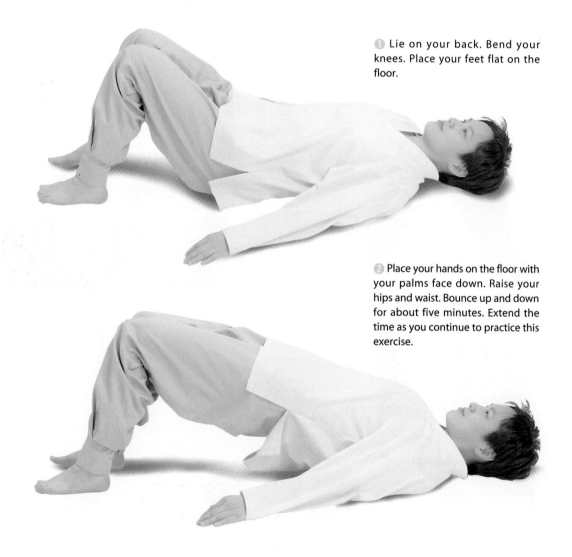

❶ Lie on your back. Bend your knees. Place your feet flat on the floor.

❷ Place your hands on the floor with your palms face down. Raise your hips and waist. Bounce up and down for about five minutes. Extend the time as you continue to practice this exercise.

3. TWISTING SIDE TO SIDE WITH KNEES BENT

TIPS   Attempt to keep your knees together when performing this exercise.

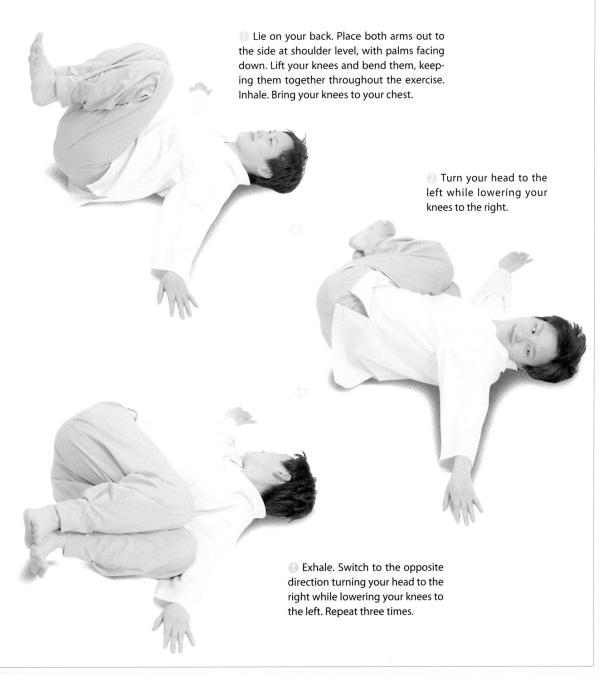

① Lie on your back. Place both arms out to the side at shoulder level, with palms facing down. Lift your knees and bend them, keeping them together throughout the exercise. Inhale. Bring your knees to your chest.

② Turn your head to the left while lowering your knees to the right.

③ Exhale. Switch to the opposite direction turning your head to the right while lowering your knees to the left. Repeat three times.

4. REALIGNING PELVIS AND WAIST

TIPS To perform this exercise correctly, it is necessary to twist your upper body in the opposite direction of your lower body.

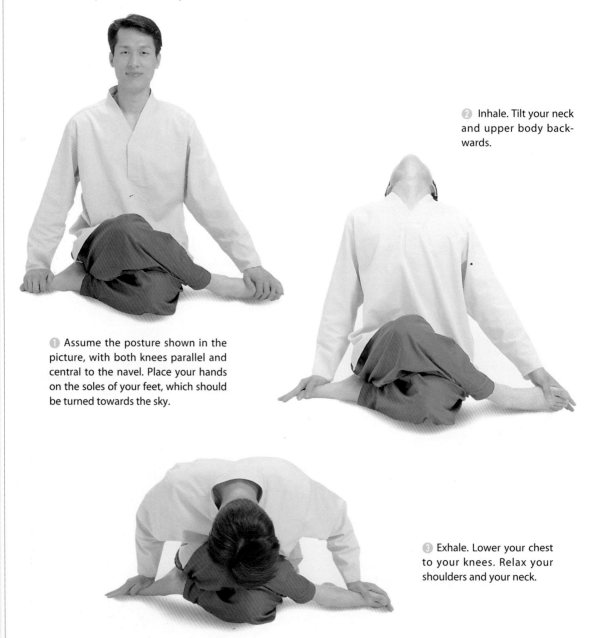

❷ Inhale. Tilt your neck and upper body backwards.

❶ Assume the posture shown in the picture, with both knees parallel and central to the navel. Place your hands on the soles of your feet, which should be turned towards the sky.

❸ Exhale. Lower your chest to your knees. Relax your shoulders and your neck.

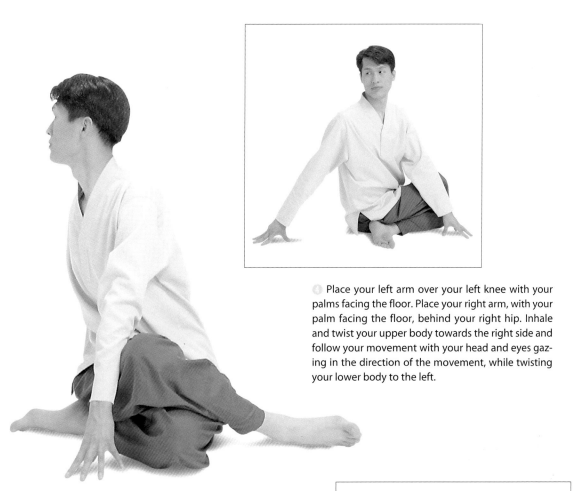

④ Place your left arm over your left knee with your palms facing the floor. Place your right arm, with your palm facing the floor, behind your right hip. Inhale and twist your upper body towards the right side and follow your movement with your head and eyes gazing in the direction of the movement, while twisting your lower body to the left.

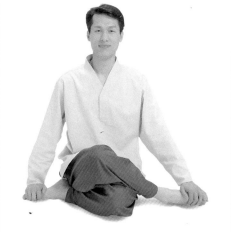

⑤ Exhale. Return to STEP1. Repeat twice. Switch positions of your legs and perform to the opposite side.

5. LYING ON YOUR STOMACH WHILE CROSSING LEGS

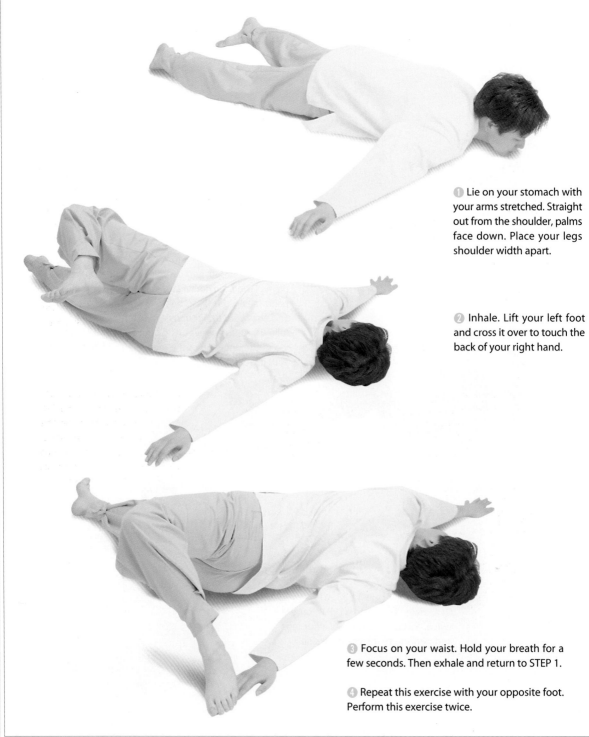

❶ Lie on your stomach with your arms stretched. Straight out from the shoulder, palms face down. Place your legs shoulder width apart.

❷ Inhale. Lift your left foot and cross it over to touch the back of your right hand.

❸ Focus on your waist. Hold your breath for a few seconds. Then exhale and return to STEP 1.

❹ Repeat this exercise with your opposite foot. Perform this exercise twice.

6. LYING lotus postion WITH OVERHEAD STRETCH

Benefits Aligns and strengthens the lumbar spine and opens the chest.

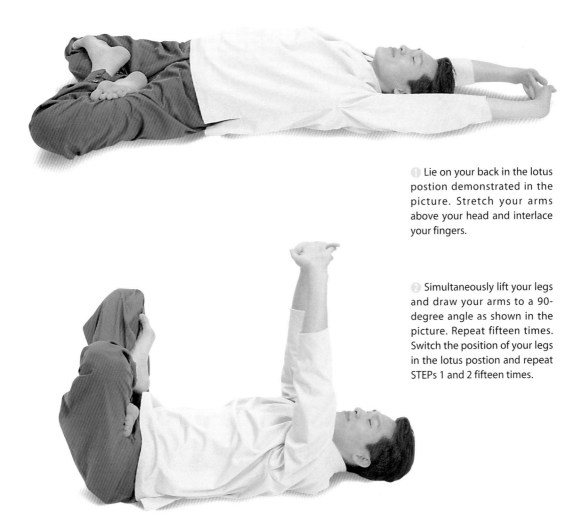

① Lie on your back in the lotus postion demonstrated in the picture. Stretch your arms above your head and interlace your fingers.

② Simultaneously lift your legs and draw your arms to a 90-degree angle as shown in the picture. Repeat fifteen times. Switch the position of your legs in the lotus postion and repeat STEPs 1 and 2 fifteen times.

7. WAGGING YOUR TAIL

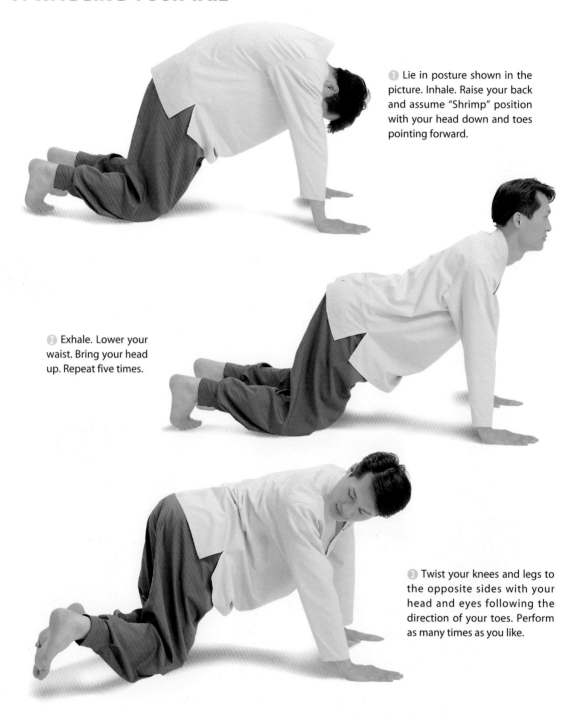

① Lie in posture shown in the picture. Inhale. Raise your back and assume "Shrimp" position with your head down and toes pointing forward.

② Exhale. Lower your waist. Bring your head up. Repeat five times.

③ Twist your knees and legs to the opposite sides with your head and eyes following the direction of your toes. Perform as many times as you like.

8. PULLING KNEES TO CHEST

TIPS Do not perform this exercise if you have been diagnosed with high blood pressure.

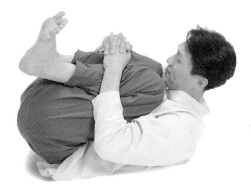

1 Lie on your back. Inhale. Bring your knees to your chest. Hold your breath. Point your toes toward your Dahn-jon, with your chin touching your knees.

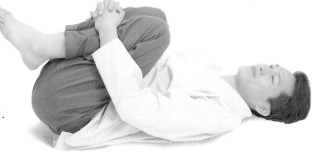

2 Exhale and return to STEP 1.

9. UPPER BODY LIFT

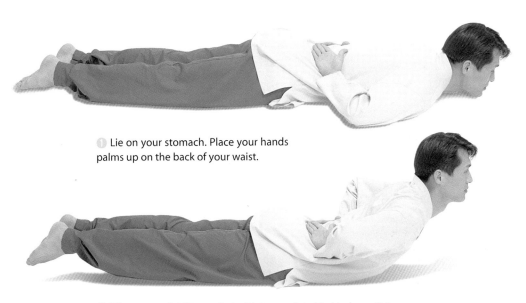

1 Lie on your stomach. Place your hands palms up on the back of your waist.

2 Lift your trunk. Lift your feet with toes pointed behind you. Return to STEP 1. Repeat twenty times.

10. SIT-UP

Benefits Exercises 9 and 10 strengthens your upper abdomen and waist, and re-aligns the lumbar spine.

TIPS Perform this exercise very slowly. Pay attention to the sensations in your waist and abdomen.

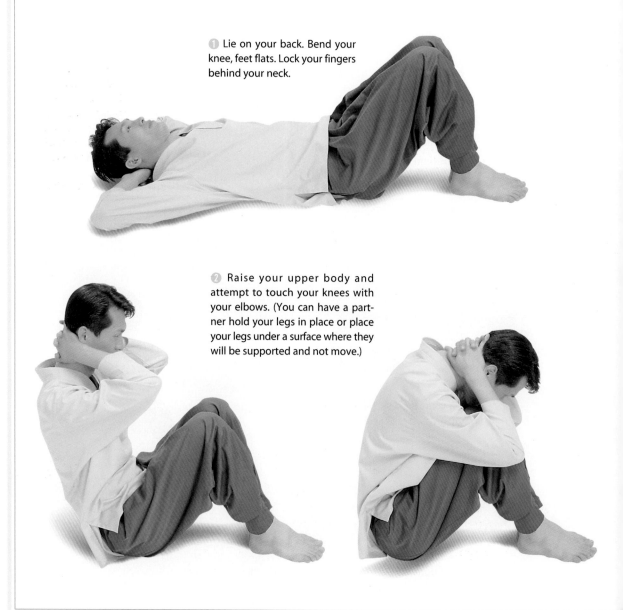

❶ Lie on your back. Bend your knee, feet flats. Lock your fingers behind your neck.

❷ Raise your upper body and attempt to touch your knees with your elbows. (You can have a partner hold your legs in place or place your legs under a surface where they will be supported and not move.)

11. HEAD-UP HANG-GONG

Benefits Beneficial for lumbago and the kidneys. Expedites Ki energy accumulation in the Dahn-jon, strengthens muscles around the waist and relieves pain in the neck and the shoulders.

TIPS If you have been diagnosed with disc problems, perform this exercise judiciously. Increase the time you maintain this posture with caution.

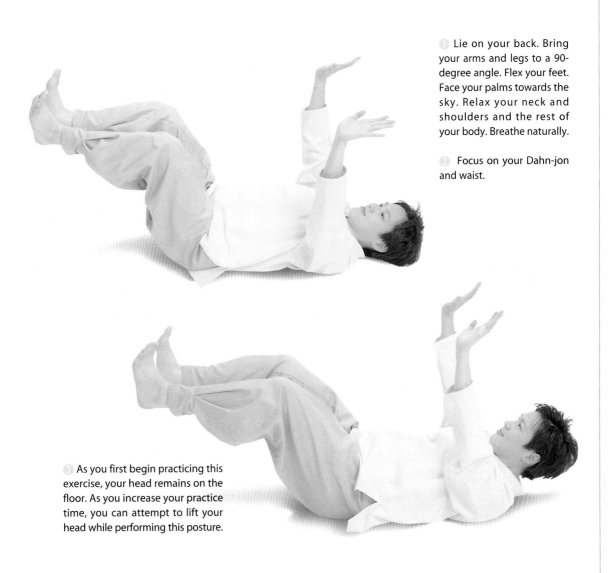

❶ Lie on your back. Bring your arms and legs to a 90-degree angle. Flex your feet. Face your palms towards the sky. Relax your neck and shoulders and the rest of your body. Breathe naturally.

❷ Focus on your Dahn-jon and waist.

❸ As you first begin practicing this exercise, your head remains on the floor. As you increase your practice time, you can attempt to lift your head while performing this posture.

2) NECK PAIN

∽

The cervical spine comprises the neck. There are seven cervical vertebrae. The neck connects the head and the body with nervous system activity through the cervical spine. Muscles surround the neck to keep it erect. When you experience pain in the neck area, the etiology is most commonly from muscular problems. Sometimes there may be a herniated or protruded disc. One of the ways to detect a disc problem is to sit in the lotus postion. Place palms on top of the head and exert pressure on the head. If you experience pain, it may signal a disc problem. Cervical misalignment or stiffness of muscles around the neck and shoulder could also be accompanied by neck pain.

If you have a diagnosed disc problem, observe yourself. Watch how your neck moves as you very slowly rotate it in different positions. Relax your neck and shoulders as you perform this. You may choose from the many postures recommened according to what is most feasible for you to do, contingent upon your particular condition. If you have a protruded or herniated disc, located either in your cervical or lumbar spine, it could signal a problem in the liver or the kidneys. Meridian exercises will help stimulate and challenge the liver, kidneys and cervical spine. If you experience neck pain, it is imperative to keep the neck warm. You may use hot compresses applied to the neck for twenty minutes at a time and then repeat the procedure.

NECK MASSAGE (p. 37)

Method When you massage your neck, you can focus on the areas where you have pain.

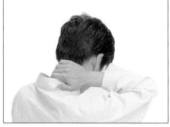

REALAXING THE TRAPEZIUS MUSCLE (p. 37)

Benefits Head, neck, shoulders, and trapezius muscle become relaxed. Massage your trapezius muscle and your shoulders.

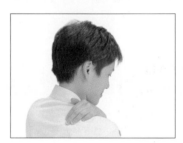

MOVING A JAR (p. 49)

Benefits Aligns the spine and rib cage. Helps relieve cervical disc problems, facial paralysis, shoulder pain, and symptoms of tuberculosis.

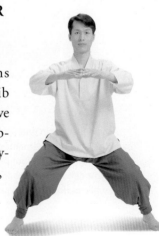

HEAD-UP HANG-GONG (p. 109)

Benefits If you raise your head, circulation in the head and neck is more efficient, relieving neck pain. This exercise also aligns the cervical spine and strengthens neck muscles.

TIPS If you have a diagnosed problem in your cervical spine, you may wish to proceed with this posture by keeping your head on the floor. Proceed with this position judiciously.

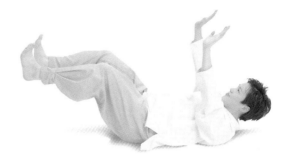

1. USING WOODEN PILLOW

Benefits This exercise expedites energy flow to the head, brain, and nervous system. It enhances mental clarity and visual acuity. It also opens acupressure points around the neck and aligns the spinal cord.

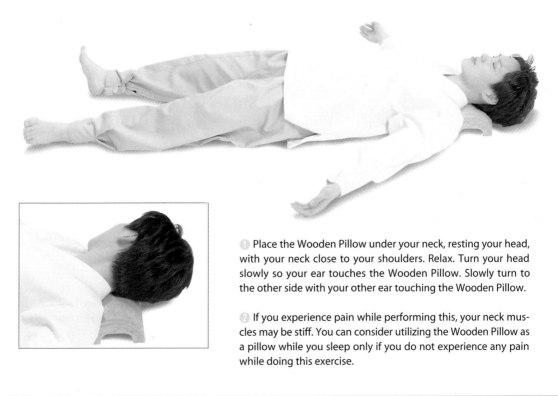

① Place the Wooden Pillow under your neck, resting your head, with your neck close to your shoulders. Relax. Turn your head slowly so your ear touches the Wooden Pillow. Slowly turn to the other side with your other ear touching the Wooden Pillow.

② If you experience pain while performing this, your neck muscles may be stiff. You can consider utilizing the Wooden Pillow as a pillow while you sleep only if you do not experience any pain while doing this exercise.

2. HEAD LIFT

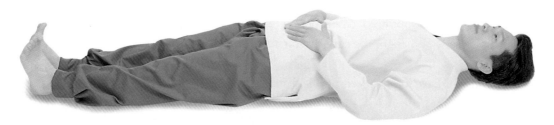

① Lie down on your back with your feet together and your toes flexed toward your body. Place your hands on your Dahn-jon.

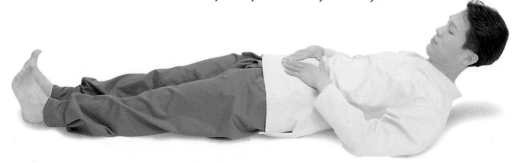

② Lift your head up and down slowly.

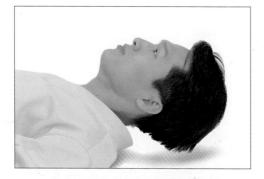

③ Continue to move your head up and down, but do not touch the floor with your head as you lower it. Repeat this twenty times.

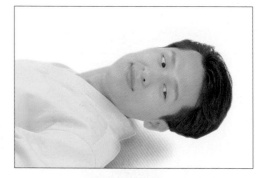

④ Lift your head up slowly and carefully. Alternate moving it left and right.

3. NECK EXERCISE

TIPS   Maintain focus on your neck as you perform these movements. Move only your neck and head very slowly. Relax the rest of your body.

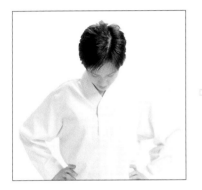 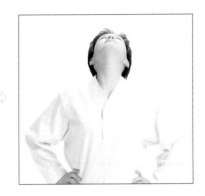

① Stand. Place your hands on your waist. Move your head very slowly in a circular motion. When you move forward, touch your chin to your chest. Breathe naturally.

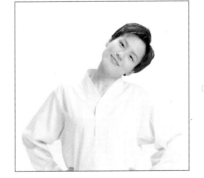 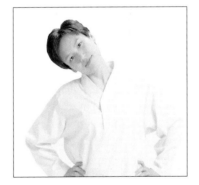

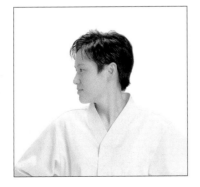

② Slowly turn your head to the left. Inhale. Hold your breath. Face forward and exhale through your mouth. As you do this, imagine the stagnant energy from your neck exiting the body through your mouth. Repeat this movement to the right.

3) SHOULDER PAIN

Pain in the shoulders is most often accompanied by stress. When you experience stress or High Blood Pressure, for example, the muscles in the shoulder can go into spasm or feel stiff. Pain in the shoulder region may also be caused by organ malfunction.

The shoulder is the conduit for the circulation of blood through the vessels and into the brain. When the muscles in the shoulder contract and become stiff, oxygen in the blood cannot pass easily to the brain, thereby depriving the brain of the necessary oxygen to be transported throughout the blood system. Oftentimes, faulty postural habits can cause shoulder misalignment.

Consequentially, the integrity of major organs, such as the lungs and heart, are compromised in their function. In Eastern Medicine, it is believed that when shoulder pain is present, blood becomes stagnant and there is a proliferation of energy blockage around the muscles of the neck and shoulder. Significant deprivation of range of motion in the shoulder with intensified pain is experienced.

When you perform the exercises recommended in this chapter, you can ultimately experience significant relief of your shoulder pain. This is because the exercises provide improved Ki energy and blood circulation, with fresh oxygen flow to nourish the muscles and release stagnant blood from the affected shoulder region.

NECK MASSAGE (p. 37)

Method In addition to self-massage, you can also ask someone to assist you in massaging the painful muscle area in the back of your neck.

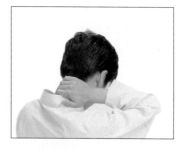

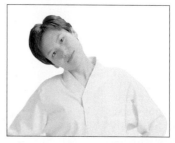

BATHING REMEDY :

- Frozen Shoulder- the ligaments of the joints become stiff around the shoulder. This discomfort can be relieved by soaking in a tub of water that is comfortably heated.
- You can stand in a pool with water at shoulder level or higher while slowly performing the breast- stroke with your arms. Enlarge the range of motion with which you perform this stroke as you progress in practice.
- Place yourself in alternating water temperature environments. For example, switch from the cool pool to a hot tub environment.
- Spend about three to four minutes in cool water and then another three to four minutes in the hot water.

1. PUSHING PALMS

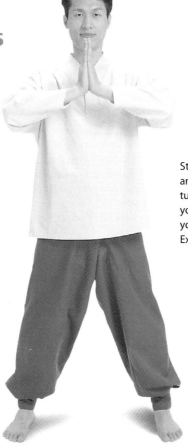

Stand with your feet shoulder width apart and your palms together as shown in the picture. Inhale. Hold your breath while you open your chest and exert pressure while pushing your palms together. Hold for a few seconds. Exhale. Repeat five times.

2. PULLING THE ELBOW BEHIND THE HEAD

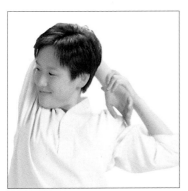
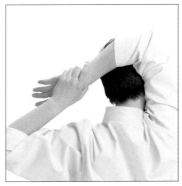
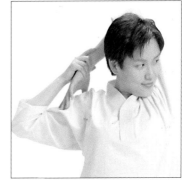

❶ Place your right elbow behind your head. Hold the wrist of your right hand with your left hand as shown in the picture. Inhale. Pull the wrist of the right hand with your left hand. Focus on your shoulder joint while you perform this exercise.

❷ Exhale. Release. Repeat twice with each arm.

3. CROSS ARMS, CLASP, and TWIST

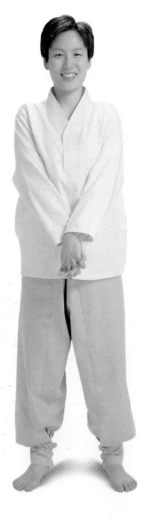

❶ Cross your arms. Lock your fingers and assume the position as in the picture. Inhale. Wrap your arms under and bring them towards your chest in a circular motion. Stretch your arms out and away from your chest and straighten your arms out in front of your body. Continuing to clasp your hands, bend your neck backwards and stretch.

❷ Hold for a few seconds. Exhale. Return to STEP 1 and repeat this exercise by switching the positions of your hands.

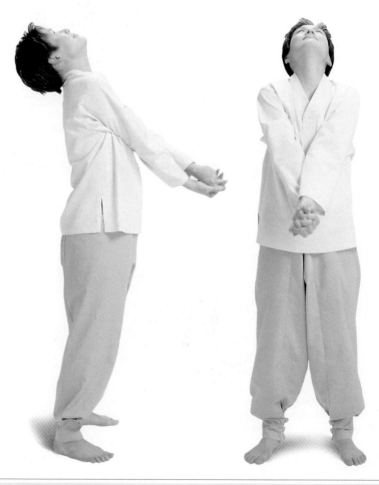

4. ROTATING ARMS

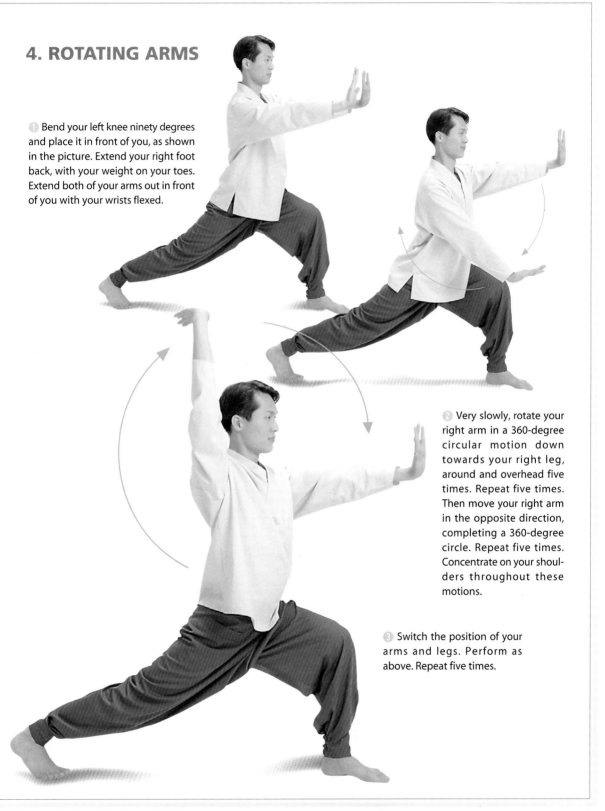

1 Bend your left knee ninety degrees and place it in front of you, as shown in the picture. Extend your right foot back, with your weight on your toes. Extend both of your arms out in front of you with your wrists flexed.

2 Very slowly, rotate your right arm in a 360-degree circular motion down towards your right leg, around and overhead five times. Repeat five times. Then move your right arm in the opposite direction, completing a 360-degree circle. Repeat five times. Concentrate on your shoulders throughout these motions.

3 Switch the position of your arms and legs. Perform as above. Repeat five times.

5. UPPER BODY BEND WITH CLASPED HANDS BEHIND BACK

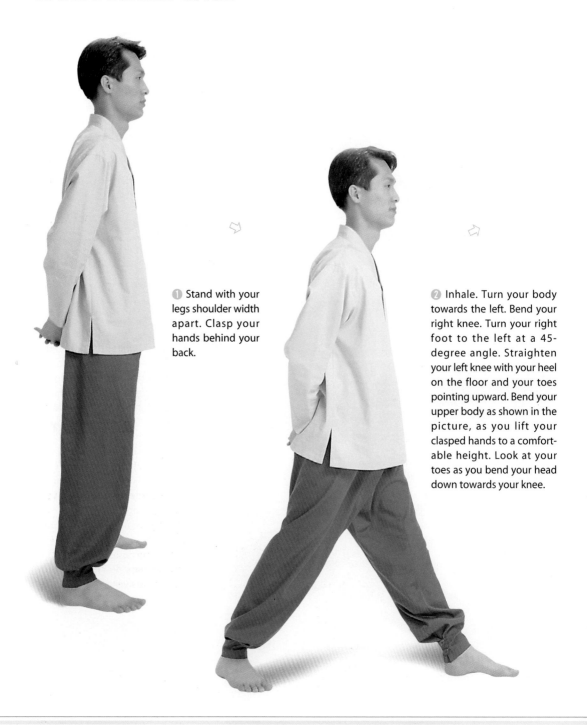

❶ Stand with your legs shoulder width apart. Clasp your hands behind your back.

❷ Inhale. Turn your body towards the left. Bend your right knee. Turn your right foot to the left at a 45-degree angle. Straighten your left knee with your heel on the floor and your toes pointing upward. Bend your upper body as shown in the picture, as you lift your clasped hands to a comfortable height. Look at your toes as you bend your head down towards your knee.

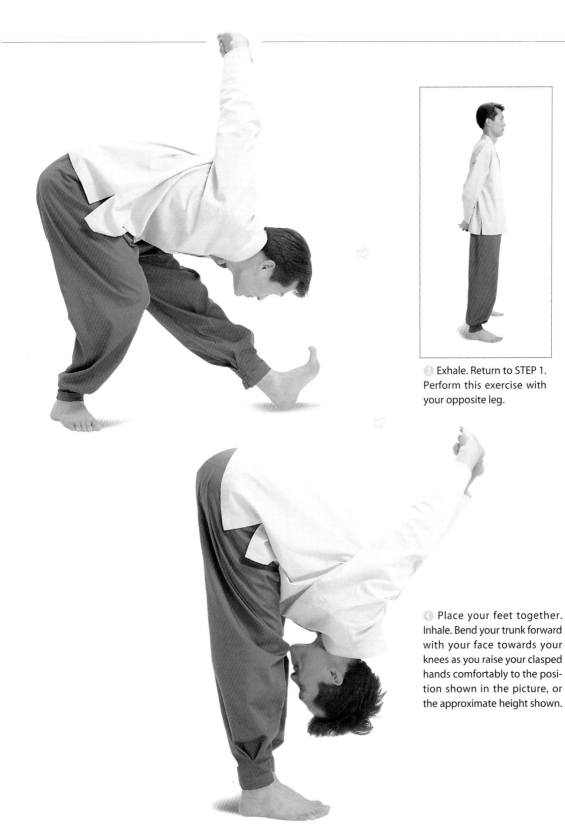

③ Exhale. Return to STEP 1. Perform this exercise with your opposite leg.

④ Place your feet together. Inhale. Bend your trunk forward with your face towards your knees as you raise your clasped hands comfortably to the position shown in the picture, or the approximate height shown.

6. CLAP HANDS

Benefits Brings heat energy around the muscles of the shoulder, as Ki energy and blood circulation is facilitated.

① Stand with your feet shoulder width apart. Place your palms touching together as shown in the picture.

② Clap your hands in front of your face, behind your head, and behind your waist, one time each. This comprises one repetition. Keep your head straight, while relaxing the muscles in your neck and shoulders. Repeat fifty times.

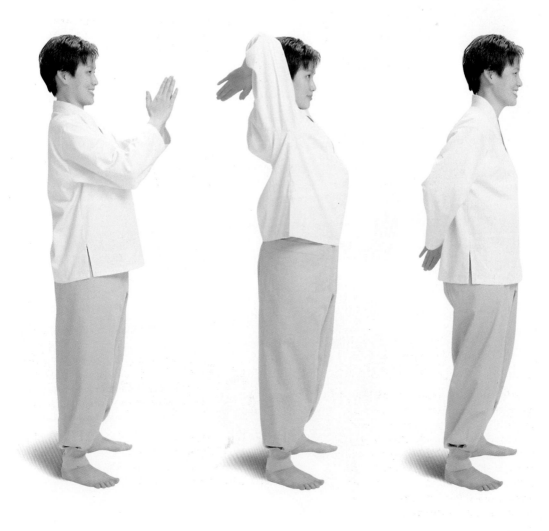

7. FORWARD BEND FOR SHOULDER

Benefits This exercise relieves tension in the shoulder muscles, hands, and arms. It rejuvenates the hand as you press with your thumb to stimulate the meridians on the back of your hand.

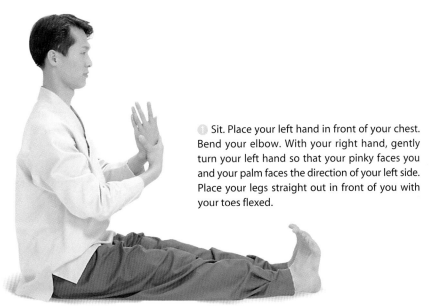

① Sit. Place your left hand in front of your chest. Bend your elbow. With your right hand, gently turn your left hand so that your pinky faces you and your palm faces the direction of your left side. Place your legs straight out in front of you with your toes flexed.

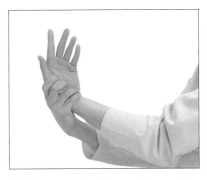

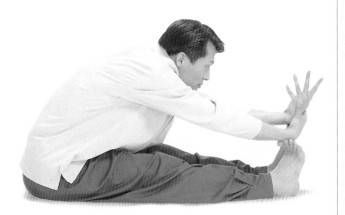

② Place your four fingers of your right hand on the pad of your left palm. Place your right thumb on the back of the left hand, as depicted in the picture. Slightly twist the left hand with your right thumb as you press into the back of your left hand with your right thumb in the position demonstrated. This acupressure position will activate several meridians.

③ Inhale. While maintaining the position of your hands, bend your trunk forward with your arms straight and touch your toes with the back of your right hand. Focus on your shoulders. Exhale and return to STEP 1.

4) SCIATIC PAIN

The Sciatic nerve is the largest of the Peripheral nerves. Sciatic pain, known as Sciatica, is experienced by most people as severe. Its origin is the lumbar spine. It radiates deeply into the muscles of the buttocks, coursing down the posterior part of each leg and through the back of the thigh and calf. In severe cases, pain radiates and extends into the foot. It can be accompanied by numbness and tingling. It can be easily palpated, which accounts for the lower threshold in response to experiencing the intense sensation of pain.

The etiology of sciatica can be multifaceted, including peripheral nerve root compression from herniated discs, weakness of the kidneys, faulty posture habits, and long-term sedentary life-styles, changes in joints due to bony growths, such as osteoarthritis, muscle spasms, and irritated tissues around the joints of the spine. In severe cases, people compensate for the pain by shifting their weight into other parts of their body, causing asymmetry and misalignment and exacerbating the problem. They will oftentimes favor the side of the body that does not experience the sciatica. It is important to maintain warmth in the lower part of the body when you experience sciatic nerve difficulty.

CLASPED HANDS FORWARD BEND (p. 81)

Method If you can, sit in half-lotus postion to perform this exercise. If you cannot assume this position, then perform with your legs crossed.

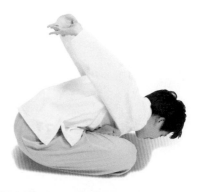

CROSSING LEGS AND TWISTING (p. 79)

Benefits This exercise relaxes knee joints, enables maximum proficiency of the autonomic nervous system, and regulates the functioning of the intestines and the accompanying organs. It promotes flexibility of the lower extremities and prevents or helps to abate neuralgia.

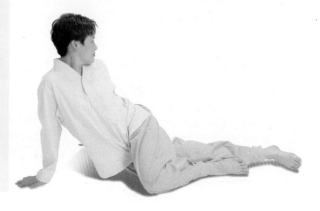

1. FOOT TO THIGH FORWARD BEND

Benefits Same as benefits of the Crossing Legs and Twisting on page 122.

TIPS Do not strain to touch your toes. Instead, reach forward and perform this exercise along the length of your leg that is most comfortably challenging.

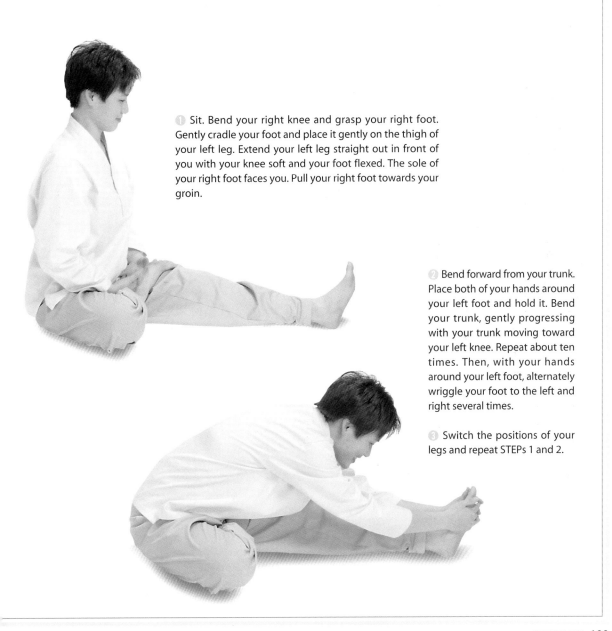

① Sit. Bend your right knee and grasp your right foot. Gently cradle your foot and place it gently on the thigh of your left leg. Extend your left leg straight out in front of you with your knee soft and your foot flexed. The sole of your right foot faces you. Pull your right foot towards your groin.

② Bend forward from your trunk. Place both of your hands around your left foot and hold it. Bend your trunk, gently progressing with your trunk moving toward your left knee. Repeat about ten times. Then, with your hands around your left foot, alternately wriggle your foot to the left and right several times.

③ Switch the positions of your legs and repeat STEPs 1 and 2.

2. REACHING PALM TOWARDS THE SKY AND TOUCHING OPPOSITE ANKLE

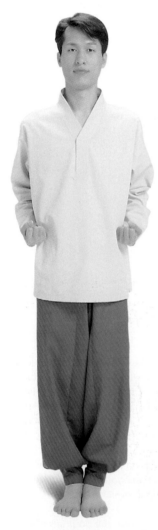

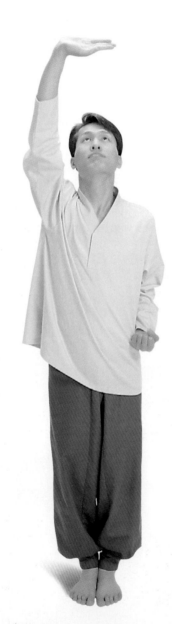

① Stand with your feet touching together. Close your hands and make fists. Place them at your sides.

② Inhale. Raise your right hand and arm with your palm facing the sky. Follow this movement of your hand with your head and eyes.

③ Hold your breath. Twist your upper body to the left.

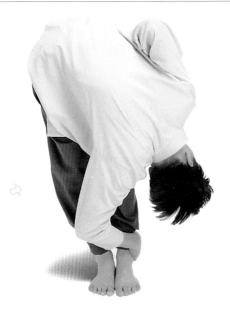

④ Bend slowly from your trunk. Grasp your left ankle with your right hand. Keep your knees straight but relaxed. Press into your ankle as you experience gentle tension. Focus on your Dahn-jon and your waist.

⑤ Exhale. Return to STEP 1 and perform to the opposite side. Repeat three times.

3. FORWARD BEND FOR WAIST AND HIPS

Benefits This exercise promotes maximum Ki energy flow to abdominal area, calms the mind, and rejuvenates the skin. It helps to prevent or abate neuralgia and promote flexibility in the knee joints.

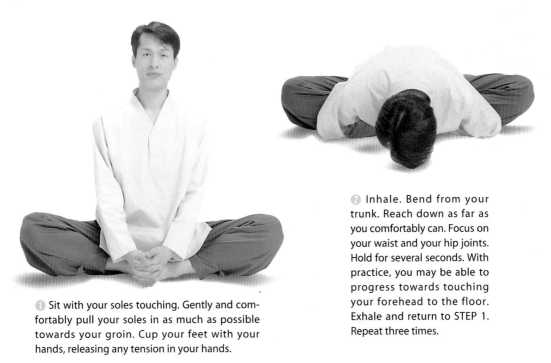

① Sit with your soles touching. Gently and comfortably pull your soles in as much as possible towards your groin. Cup your feet with your hands, releasing any tension in your hands.

② Inhale. Bend from your trunk. Reach down as far as you comfortably can. Focus on your waist and your hip joints. Hold for several seconds. With practice, you may be able to progress towards touching your forehead to the floor. Exhale and return to STEP 1. Repeat three times.

4. BENDING UPPER BODY WITH PRAYER HANDS TO THE TOES

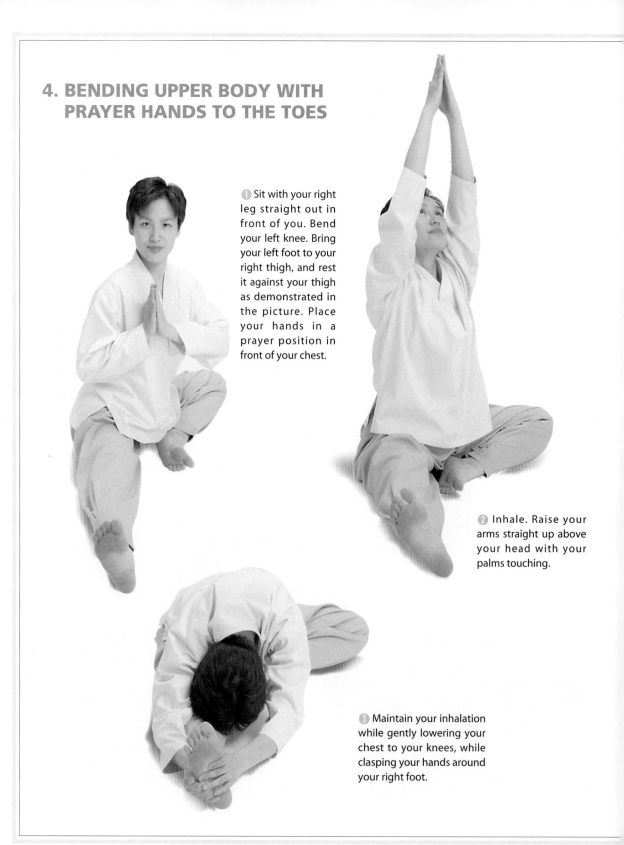

① Sit with your right leg straight out in front of you. Bend your left knee. Bring your left foot to your right thigh, and rest it against your thigh as demonstrated in the picture. Place your hands in a prayer position in front of your chest.

② Inhale. Raise your arms straight up above your head with your palms touching.

③ Maintain your inhalation while gently lowering your chest to your knees, while clasping your hands around your right foot.

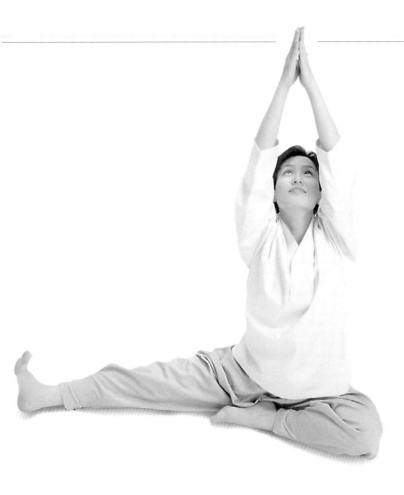

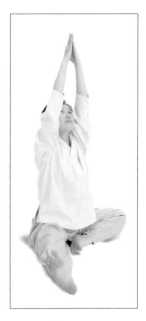

④ Return to STEP 1. Inhale. Place your palms together above your head.

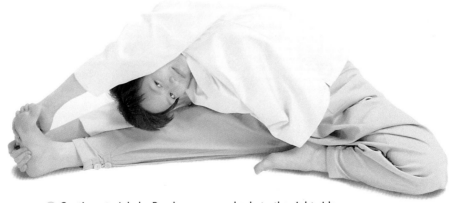

⑤ Continue to Inhale. Bend your upper body to the right side. Touch your knees with your head and look towards the sky. Place your hands around your right foot in the position depicted in the diagram.

⑥ Exhale. Return to STEP 1. Switch legs and repeat.

5. THIGH STRETCH

Benefits This exercise generates and enhances nervous system functioning from the waist to the legs and hip joints as they are relaxed and thighs are stretched. It also alleviates pain.

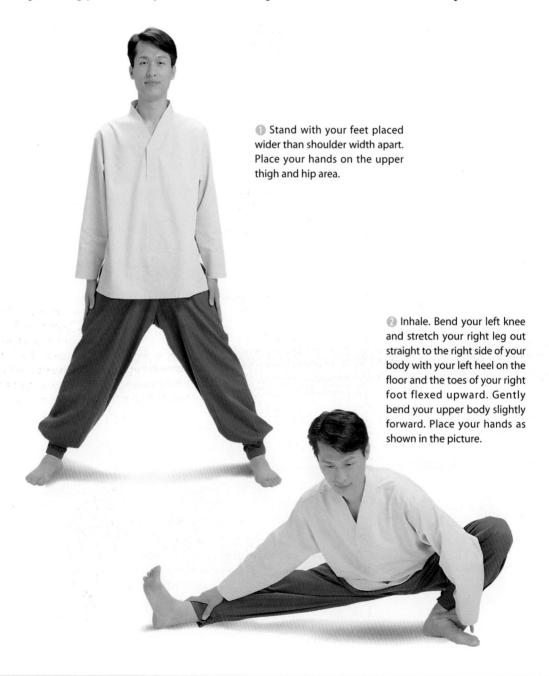

❶ Stand with your feet placed wider than shoulder width apart. Place your hands on the upper thigh and hip area.

❷ Inhale. Bend your left knee and stretch your right leg out straight to the right side of your body with your left heel on the floor and the toes of your right foot flexed upward. Gently bend your upper body slightly forward. Place your hands as shown in the picture.

③ Maintain your inhalation while bending your upper body. Turn your upper body toward your right leg with your forehead toward your right knee and your right hand holding your right ankle. Wrap your left hand around your left ankle. Exhale. Return to STEP 1. Repeat this to the opposite side.

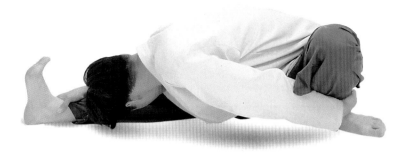

④ Turn your upper body to the left. Bend your left knee 90-degrees and place your left hand on your left thigh. Place your right hand on the back of your right thigh.

⑤ Inhale. Maintain the position of your hands from STEP 4. Open your chest. Tilt your head backwards. Raise your right heel off the floor keeping your right leg straight. Focus on your thighs and calves.

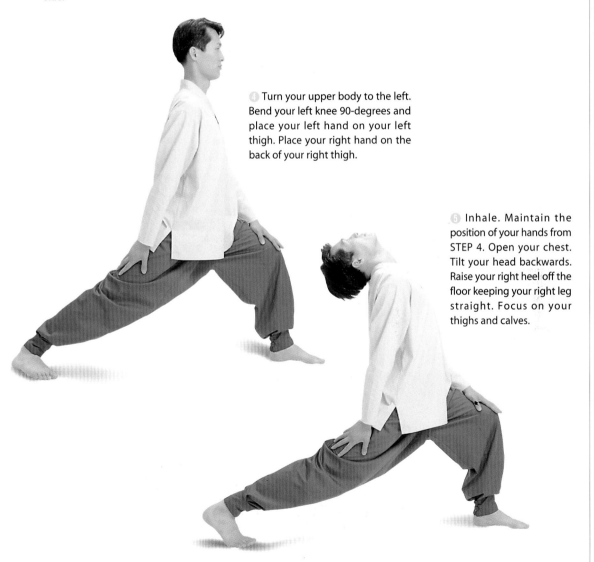

5) ARTHRITIS

The term arthritis technically refers to joint inflammation. There are several types of arthritis. This chapter will describe the two most prevalent forms: rheumatoid and degenerative arthritis. rheumatoid arthritis is the most frequently diagnosed incapacitating forms of arthritis. It is an autoimmune disease resulting from the immune system launching an assault upon the joints, rendering inflammation, stiffness, pain, redness, swelling, and heat at the site. rheumatoid arthritis can affect the body systemically, including the organs and muscles. This is due to the toxins, which accumulate as a result of prolonged inflammation.

Degenerative joint disease, or osteoarthritis, is a form of arthritis usually associated with aging. Those with this disease experience stiffness and decreased range of motion. The progression of this disease occurs as the tissue, known as the articular cartilage, lodged or nestled between the bones that comprise the joints, deteriorate and erode. Bony growths can occur with hard nodules, which differ from the more soft and spongy inflammation in the joint of someone with rheumatoid arthritis. Knees and hips are frequently attacked by degenerative joint disease because of the weight these joints must bear. The knee joint must be able to support the weight of the upper body. Ki energy and blood circulation in this joint becomes compromised and restricted. The six major joints, including the arm, elbow, wrists, knees, hips, and ankles, are vulnerable targets for arthritis, and the prime locations where energy blockages are facilitated. Unfortunately, when a person experiences pain from the inflammation, the proclivity is to avoid movement, which creates a vicious cycle, immobilizing the joint and ultimately limiting its function. To maximize the restoration of movement, energy blockages must be released to re-enable function. Ki energy and blood circulation must be augmented. The exercises in this chapter are designed to promote this process. As with any other diagnosed condition discussed in this book, consultation with an entrusted health care person with whom you can collaborate in your holistic health care is advisable.

Dahnhak Meridian exercises can help to manage the experience of the sensation of pain and discomfort in relation to arthritis. They can be utilized both as a prophylactic, as well as a palliative measure. Progressive inflammation of the joints can be deterred. As Ki energy and blood circulation freely migrate throughout your system, flexibility and strength of muscles and ligaments can be refined, with attendant increase in range of motion, so the joints around which they envelop can be protected. Impact on joints is significantly minimized and a sense of well-being is felt as you integrate and synchronize conscious breathing with your movements.

FORWARD BEND FOR WAIST AND HIPS (p. 75)

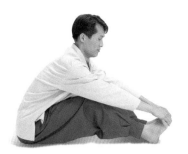

Benefits It stimulates the functioning of the kidneys and joints, including knee joints, and helps alleviate shoulder pain.

1. RELEASING HAMSTRING MUSCLES

Benefits When there are knee problems, stagnant energy lodges behind the knees. This exercise releases stagnant Ki energy from behind the knees. Ki and blood circulation is facilitated and knee joints are nourished.

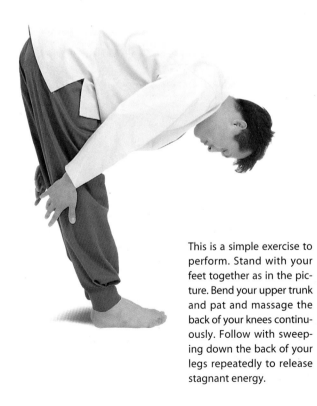

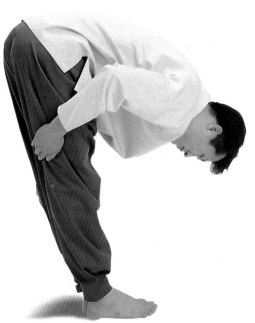

This is a simple exercise to perform. Stand with your feet together as in the picture. Bend your upper trunk and pat and massage the back of your knees continuously. Follow with sweeping down the back of your legs repeatedly to release stagnant energy.

2. KNEE FLEXION AND EXTENSION

TIPS When you exhale, imagine that you are releasing stagnant energy from your knees and sending it out through your toes.

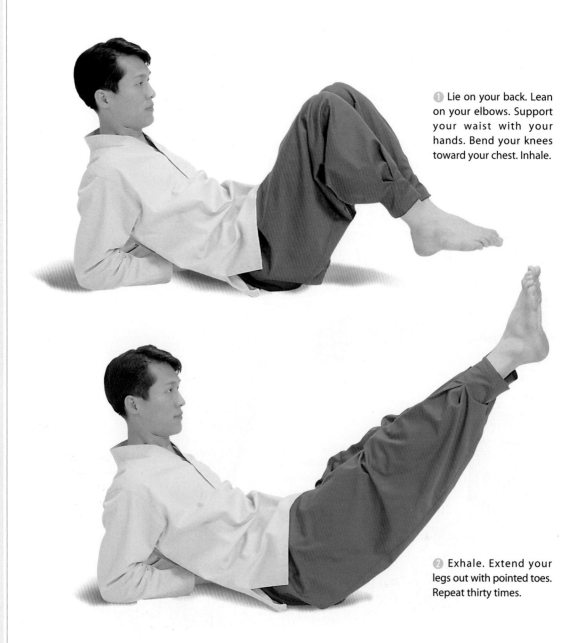

① Lie on your back. Lean on your elbows. Support your waist with your hands. Bend your knees toward your chest. Inhale.

② Exhale. Extend your legs out with pointed toes. Repeat thirty times.

3. KNEE MASSAGE WITH KI ENERGY

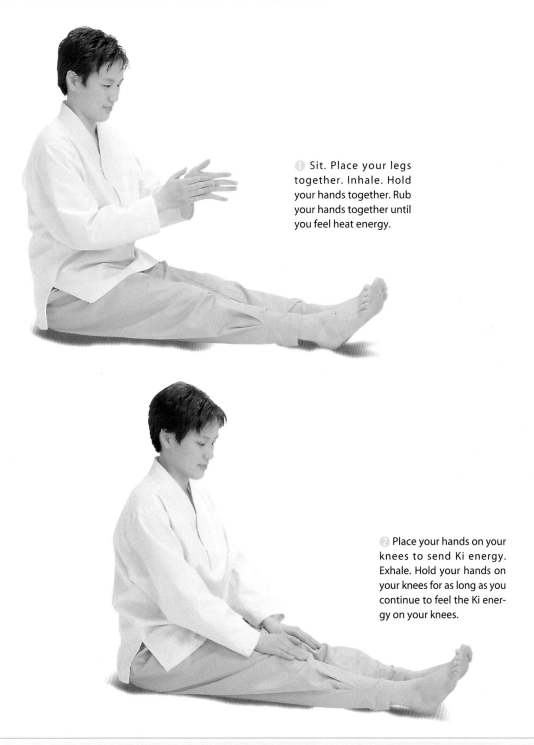

❶ Sit. Place your legs together. Inhale. Hold your hands together. Rub your hands together until you feel heat energy.

❷ Place your hands on your knees to send Ki energy. Exhale. Hold your hands on your knees for as long as you continue to feel the Ki energy on your knees.

4. KNEE EXERCISE

TIPS Keep your back relaxed and elongated with feet parallel to your shoulders. Concentrate on your knees. Repeat this exercise five times. Increase the length of time as you progress in your practice.

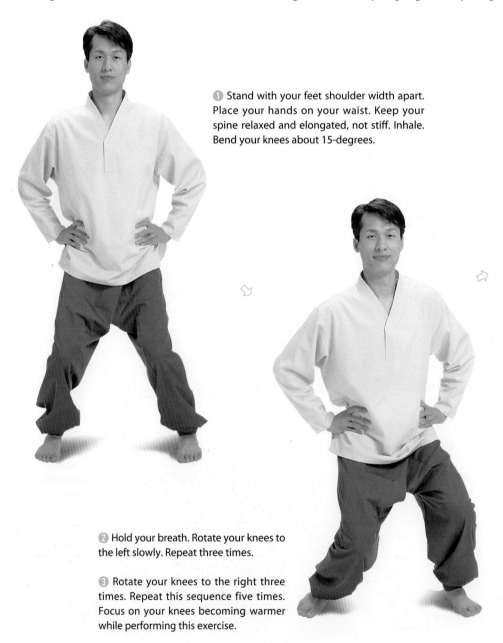

1 Stand with your feet shoulder width apart. Place your hands on your waist. Keep your spine relaxed and elongated, not stiff. Inhale. Bend your knees about 15-degrees.

2 Hold your breath. Rotate your knees to the left slowly. Repeat three times.

3 Rotate your knees to the right three times. Repeat this sequence five times. Focus on your knees becoming warmer while performing this exercise.

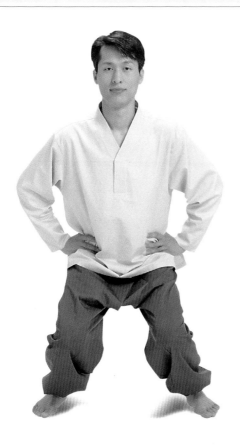

④ Inhale. Increase the bend of your knees. Hold this position for as long as comfortable. Exhale. Repeat fifteen times and return to standing.

5. HANG-GONG FOR ARTHRITIS

Benefits Knees become warmer, hip joints relax, and stagnant energy exits your lower extremities. Ki energy and blood circulation of lower extremities is facilitated.

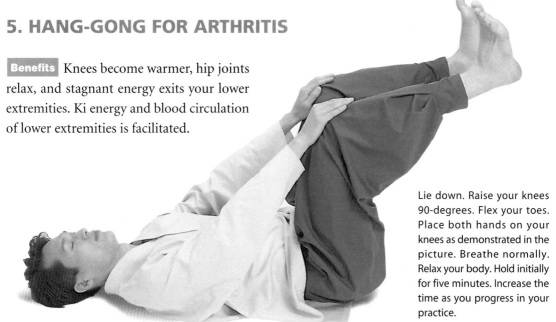

Lie down. Raise your knees 90-degrees. Flex your toes. Place both hands on your knees as demonstrated in the picture. Breathe normally. Relax your body. Hold initially for five minutes. Increase the time as you progress in your practice.

4. BONE, MUSCLE, AND SKIN

6) OSTEOPOROSIS

Osteoporosis is a condition that occurs when calcium dwindles and is leached from the bones, causing them to become porous and brittle. Bone density becomes compromised. Bones and muscles become frail and could become damaged as it becomes increasingly difficult to bear the pressure from weight-bearing daily life activities.

Symptoms of osteoporosis occur most frequently in mid-life and for women after menopause as hormone shifts occur. People oftentimes report low back pain and muscle spasms. As this disease progresses, the spine can become deformed and there is shrinkage of height. Bones can break quite easily. It is not advisable to jump or engage in any extreme movement, because the impact agitates and shocks the knee and hip joints.

SIT-UP (p. 108)

TIPS Perform this exercise slowly and focus on the movement of your body.

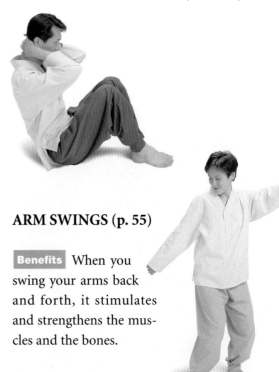

ARM SWINGS (p. 55)

Benefits When you swing your arms back and forth, it stimulates and strengthens the muscles and the bones.

STRADDLE WIHT FORWARD BEND (p. 53)

Benefits This exercise aligns pelvis and strengthens organs and bones.

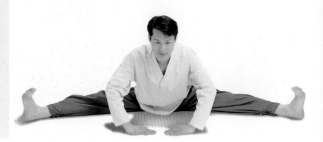

1. STANDING BODY VIBRATION

Benefits This exercise prevents and alleviates the symptoms of osteoporosis by providing deep blood and Ki energy circulation to nourish the bone marrow. It also strengthens bones and blood vessels.

① Stand with your legs shoulder width apart. Place your hands in front of you with your palms facing each other at waist level as depicted in the picture.

② Relax your whole body. Keep your fingers straight. Begin to shake your hands and arms. Imagine the vibration coursing through your entire body and notice your body begin to vibrate as well.

③ Imagine the vibration that you allow to happen, flow through the depth of every single cell from the top of your head down to your toes, nourishing, revitalizing, energizing, and healing you. Vibrate for five minutes to start and increase time with practice.

2. PUSH-UP

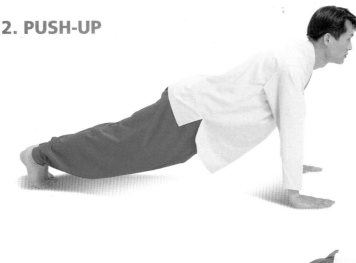

① Assume the position in the picture. Keep your spine elongated and relaxed. Face your toes towards your head. Relax your body. Bend your arms and release your chest towards the floor. Increase the time with practice.

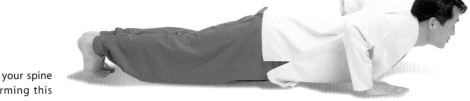

② Focus on your spine while performing this exercise.

4. BONE, MUSCLE, AND SKIN

7) SKIN DISORDERS

Scabs, dark skin pigmentations, and other skin maladies can arise often from toxins lodged in the intestines. When the intestines are functioning smoothly, problems can be eradicated, resulting in radiant and healthy skin. When you perform the recommended Intestine Exercise, along with massage of the face, ears, and areas of the head, fresh, clean, oxygenated blood and Ki energy circulation is facilitated to these areas, nourishing the tissues and nerves and cells of the skin.

When your lower extremities are raised, such that your legs are higher than your head, blood flow is expedited to the head and face. The toxins that have accumulated in the liver and kidneys can be filtered and excreted from the body. Hormonal and chemical balance is established through this self-healing intervention, thus enabling a more radiant complexion.

HEADSTAND (p. 36)

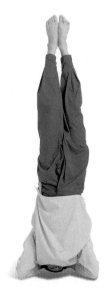

Method Beginners can try this posture against a wall for more support. As you progress, you may want to attempt this without using the wall. Begin by holding this stance for two minutes. Progress to ten minutes with practice.

TIPS If you have hypertension, heart disease, or glaucoma, it is recommended that you avoid this posture.

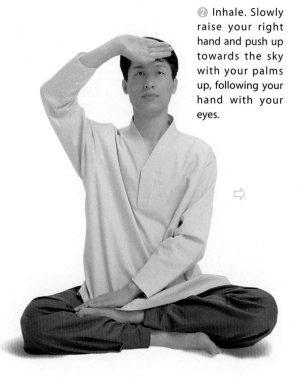

❷ Inhale. Slowly raise your right hand and push up towards the sky with your palms up, following your hand with your eyes.

1. PUSHING WITH ONE HAND ABOVE HEAD

Benefits This exercise reduces heat energy to the neck and face(as in blushing). It helps pneumonia, bronchitis, palpitations, and other upper respiratory disorders.

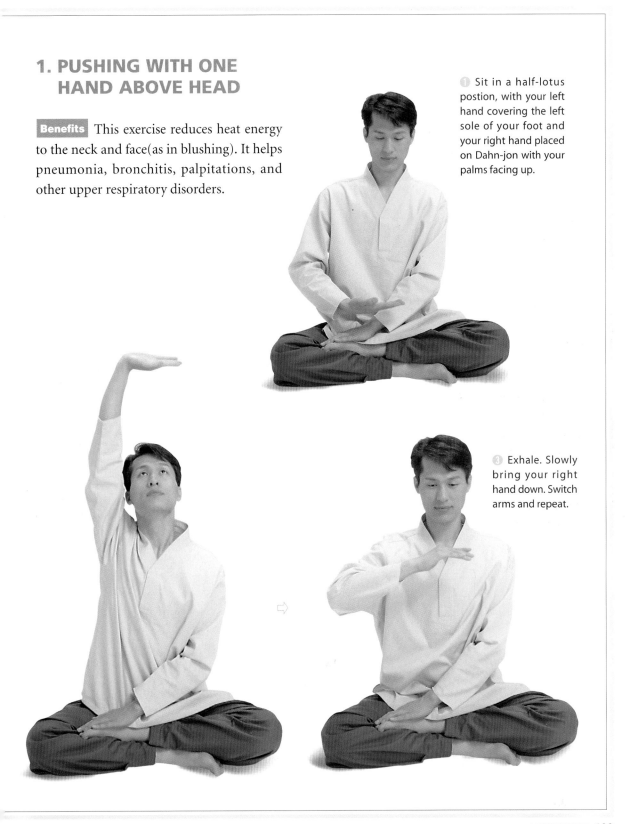

❶ Sit in a half-lotus postion, with your left hand covering the left sole of your foot and your right hand placed on Dahn-jon with your palms facing up.

❸ Exhale. Slowly bring your right hand down. Switch arms and repeat.

2. LYING LEG ROTATION

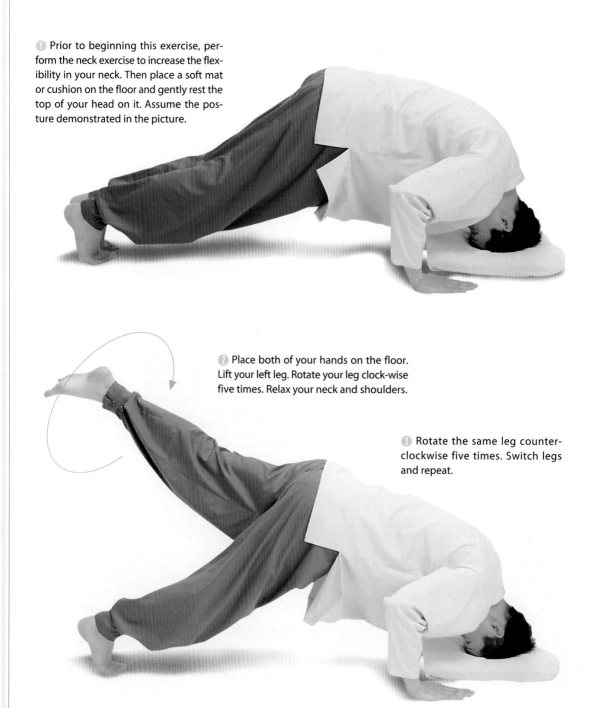

❶ Prior to beginning this exercise, perform the neck exercise to increase the flexibility in your neck. Then place a soft mat or cushion on the floor and gently rest the top of your head on it. Assume the posture demonstrated in the picture.

❷ Place both of your hands on the floor. Lift your left leg. Rotate your leg clock-wise five times. Relax your neck and shoulders.

❸ Rotate the same leg counter-clockwise five times. Switch legs and repeat.

3. SWEEPING FACE

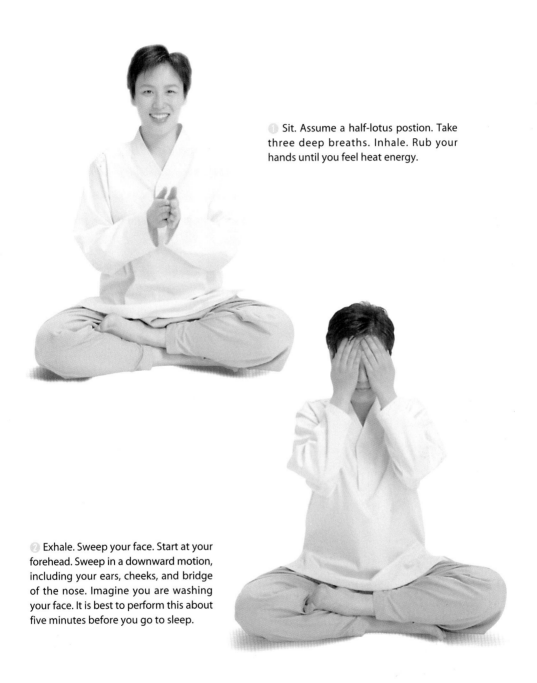

① Sit. Assume a half-lotus postion. Take three deep breaths. Inhale. Rub your hands until you feel heat energy.

② Exhale. Sweep your face. Start at your forehead. Sweep in a downward motion, including your ears, cheeks, and bridge of the nose. Imagine you are washing your face. It is best to perform this about five minutes before you go to sleep.

4. BICYCLE EXERCISE

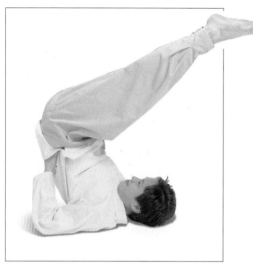

① Lie on your back. Raise both of your legs along with your upper trunk.

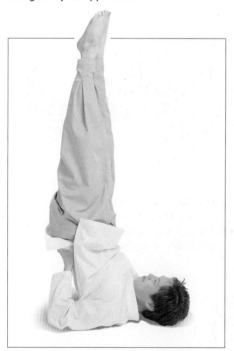

② Support your waist with both hands. Straighten your legs as shown in the picture. Keep you knees soft.

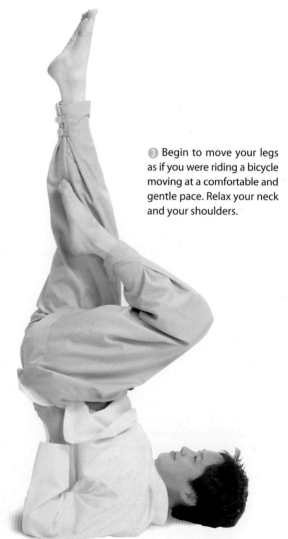

③ Begin to move your legs as if you were riding a bicycle moving at a comfortable and gentle pace. Relax your neck and your shoulders.

5. EXERCISE FOR HAIR

TIPS   You will achieve more beneficial results from this exercise the longer you are able to maintain the bending position. This exercise appears very simple, but it is challenging to execute. It is important to progress slowly, gently, comfortably, and at your own pace. As you continue to practice, you will notice you can extend your bending time, as well as reach further with more comfort.

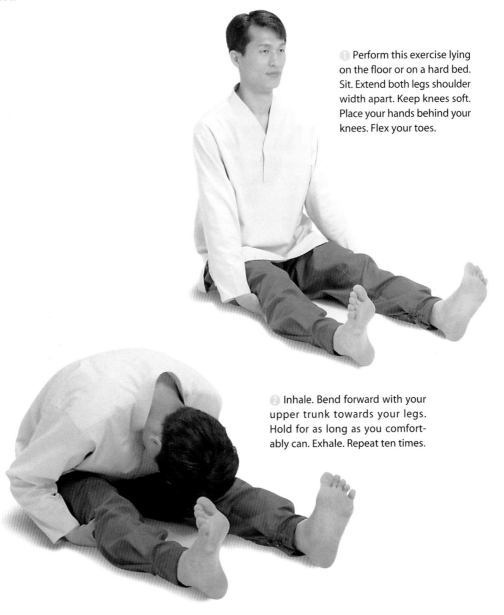

① Perform this exercise lying on the floor or on a hard bed. Sit. Extend both legs shoulder width apart. Keep knees soft. Place your hands behind your knees. Flex your toes.

② Inhale. Bend forward with your upper trunk towards your legs. Hold for as long as you comfortably can. Exhale. Repeat ten times.

6. EXERCISE TO REDUCE ITCHING

Benefits This exercise helps blood and Ki energy circulation of the shoulder and the back. Releases pain from the neck, shoulders, and arms, and relieves discomfort in the ears. It also alleviates itchiness.

TIPS It is important to extend your arms and pull them back as much as possible to open the chest and to keep your spine extended but not rigid.

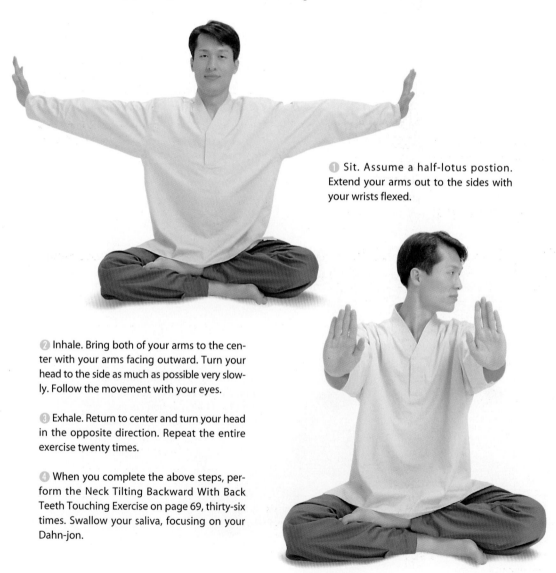

① Sit. Assume a half-lotus postion. Extend your arms out to the sides with your wrists flexed.

② Inhale. Bring both of your arms to the center with your arms facing outward. Turn your head to the side as much as possible very slowly. Follow the movement with your eyes.

③ Exhale. Return to center and turn your head in the opposite direction. Repeat the entire exercise twenty times.

④ When you complete the above steps, perform the Neck Tilting Backward With Back Teeth Touching Exercise on page 69, thirty-six times. Swallow your saliva, focusing on your Dahn-jon.

7. FACE REJUVENATION

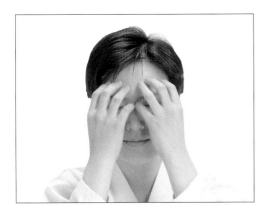

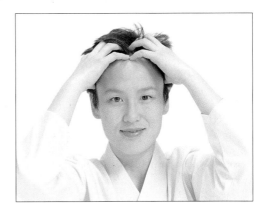

① Sit on the floor. Place your fingers on your forehead. Gently perform a raking and massaging movement down towards your eyebrows.

② Repeat this in the opposite direction moving from your eyebrows upward, including the circumference of your head.

8. NOSE LIFT EXERCISE

TIPS   This exercise is best done before going to sleep because it can cause redness around the nose.

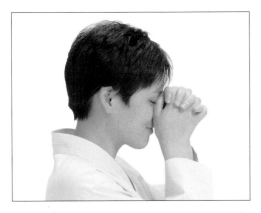

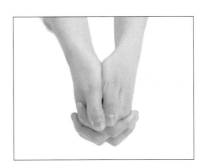

Lock your fingers. Raise them towards your nose with the pads of your hands. Encircle the nose. Pull forward on the cartilage of the nose and repeat this for two minutes. You will notice the effects of this exercise if you practice daily after about one or two months.

9. FACE UP UPPER BODY LIFT

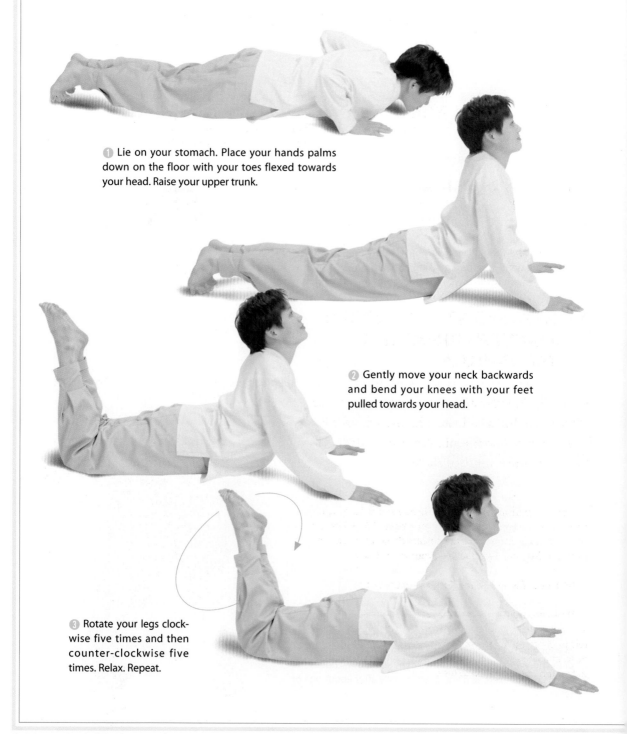

❶ Lie on your stomach. Place your hands palms down on the floor with your toes flexed towards your head. Raise your upper trunk.

❷ Gently move your neck backwards and bend your knees with your feet pulled towards your head.

❸ Rotate your legs clockwise five times and then counter-clockwise five times. Relax. Repeat.

10. SMOOTHING EYE WRINKLES

Benefits Supplies moisture to the skin around the eyes by enhancing the blood and Ki energy circulation to this area.

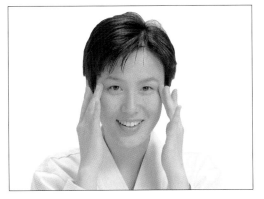

Place your middle finger on your temples. Massage with a circular motion until the area feels moist.

11. HEALING SKIN DISORDERS THROUGH BREATHING TECHNIQUES

Benefits The relaxation of the body and calming of the mind that is promoted through this exercise, when practiced twenty minutes or more daily, will assist in improving skin disorders.

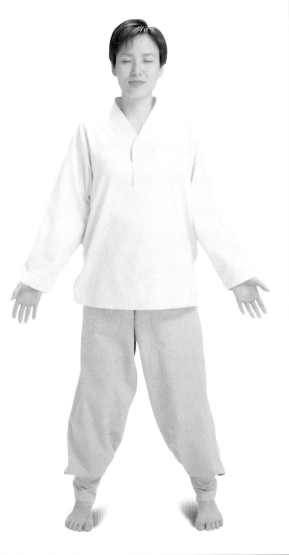

1 You can perform this exercise while standing or lying down. If you are standing, bend your knees 15-degrees. If you are lying down, assume the posture demonstrated in the picture. Close your eyes and relax your whole body.

2 Breathe softly and gently. Focus on your mind.

3 When you exhale, imagine that your approximately 84,000 skin pores will open and stagnant energy will thereby be released through these pores. When you inhale through your nose, imagine allowing fresh Ki energy to circulate throughout your body from head to toes.

4. BONE, MUSCLE, AND SKIN

8) HAIR LOSS

The medical term for hair loss is alopecia. Under normal circumstances, people lose on the average seventy to eighty hairs daily. If hair loss is in excess of this, you may be experiencing alopecia. Hair loss can result from pulling on our hair, braiding the hair, or brushing it roughly. Six weeks to three months following a high fever, you may notice hair loss. Medications you take for thyroid disorders, heart disease, cancer, and arthritis may result in hair loss as well. In addition, hair loss may occur two to three months following major surgical intervention, as well as post-natally. Stress and emotional disorders exacerbate the probability of hair loss. It is believed in Eastern Medicine that hair loss is related to kidney dysfunction. If you have normal or active kidney function, which is accompanied by heightened stamina, this will be reflected in healthy hair.

Practicing Dahn-jon breathing will act to inhibit accelerated aging. Healthy hair is augmented, as cells are rejuvenated. It is recommended that you supplement the exercises in this section with exercises that promote healthy kidney functioning.

SITTING FORWARD BEND (p. 52)

Benefits This strengthens kidney functioning and treats alopecia, promoting healthy hair.

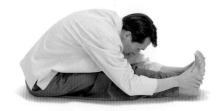

1. LYING ON YOUR BACK WITH KNEES BENT

Assume the posture demonstrated in the picture. Soles are face up, palms are face down, and fingers are facing the feet.

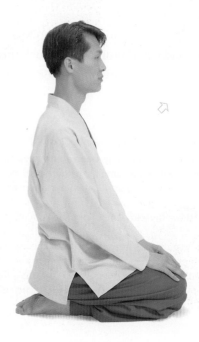

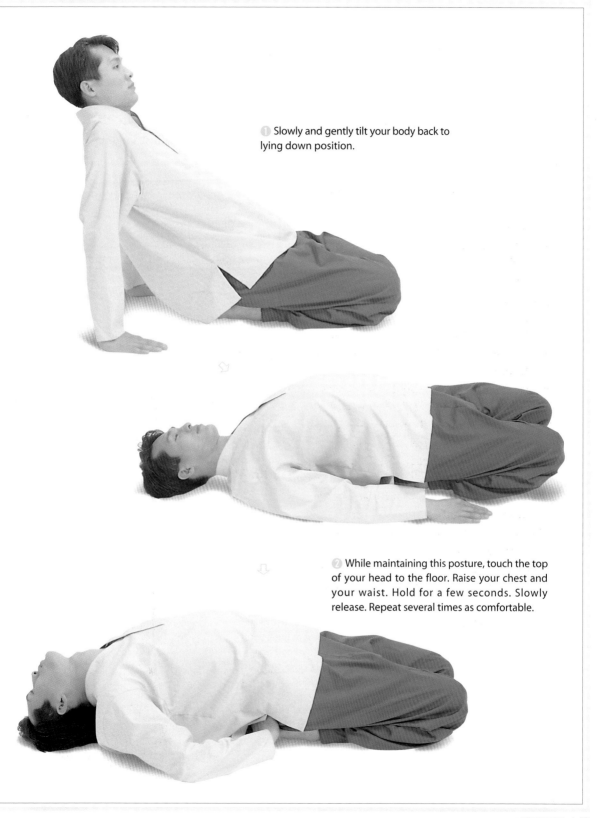

① Slowly and gently tilt your body back to lying down position.

② While maintaining this posture, touch the top of your head to the floor. Raise your chest and your waist. Hold for a few seconds. Slowly release. Repeat several times as comfortable.

2. HEAD TAPPING AND COMBING WITH FINGERTIPS

Benefits If there is not sufficient blood and Ki energy circulation to the scalp, dandruff and other dermatological disturbances and viral disorders to the scalp may occur. This can result in hair loss. Stimulating the scalp with tapping will strengthen hair roots and result in hair luster.

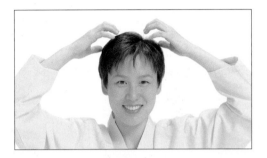

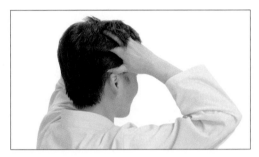

① Using your fingertips, gently tap the circumference of the head. If you have damaged or brittle hair, or if your hair breaks easily, tap very lightly.

② Using your fingertips, begin at the hair line around the ears and gently, in a raking or combing motion, move up towards the top and circumference of your head. Gently move from the hairline on the top of your forehead to the top of the head and then to the back of the head. Also, move to the hairline at the back of the neck and comb or rake up towards the top of the head. Focus on your scalp and the calming of the mind that can occur from this massage.

3. CURLING INTO A BALL

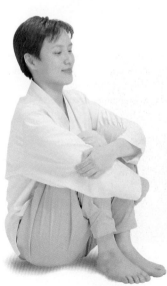

① Sit. Place your feet flat on the floor. Embrace your knees with both of your arms. Inhale. Focus on your Dahn-jon. Gently pull your knees toward your chest while simultaneously bending from your trunk to enable your chest to meet your knees. Lower your head gently to touch your face to your knees.

② Hold for a few seconds. Relax your body. Exhale and release. Repeat as often as you are comfortable.

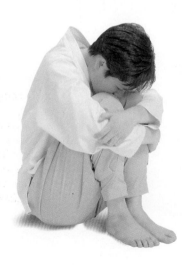

4. EXERCISE FOR HAIR LOSS

Benefits This exercise promotes blood and Ki energy circulation to the head while strengthening the functioning of the kidneys.

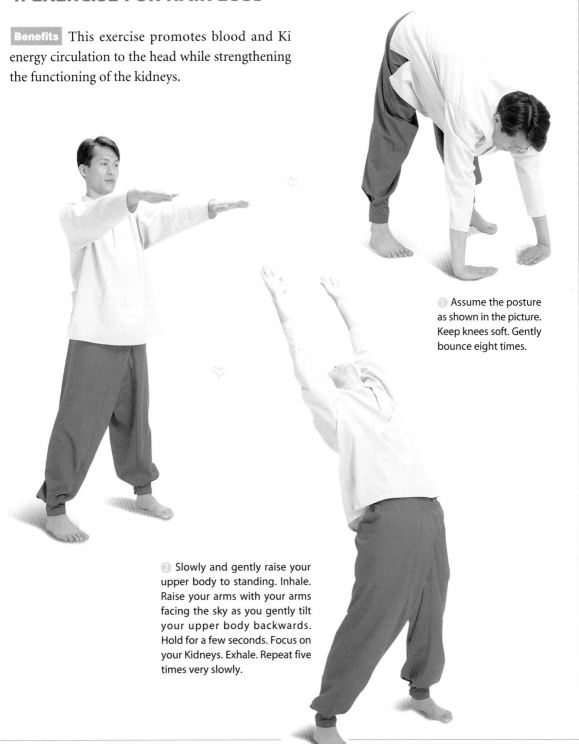

① Assume the posture as shown in the picture. Keep knees soft. Gently bounce eight times.

② Slowly and gently raise your upper body to standing. Inhale. Raise your arms with your arms facing the sky as you gently tilt your upper body backwards. Hold for a few seconds. Focus on your Kidneys. Exhale. Repeat five times very slowly.